John Stirling came to New Zealand from Britain in 1947 after service in the Royal Army Veterinary Corps. He graduated from the Royal (Dick) Veterinary College in Edinburgh in 1944, before joining the Army and serving in India, the U.K. and Germany. He was demobbed as a Major in 1947.

Soon after demobilisation he arrived in New Zealand and was located at Ohaeawai. He was the first vet to engage in general practice in the middle and far north of the North Island. This resulted in all sorts of veterinary and other adventures through the years. Later he was involved in government service both in the field and within the Meat Division of the Department of Agriculture, while concurrently running his own practice.

Turning to farming he founded the *Cairnhill* Friesian stud and *Carnbroe* Hereford stud. He was also a member of the National Hydatids Council, the N.Z. Veterinary Association, and a foundation member of the Australian College of Veterinary Scientists.

John Stirling now lives in Whangarei where he writes a monthly column for the Nor*thern Advocate*. He is presently working on a collection of short stories as a successor to his first book *On Four Legs and Two*.

For the Family

From the Hills Above Taiamai

by John Stirling

Illustrated by Bob Darroch

BENTON-GUY PUBLISHING
Box 8569, Symonds Street, Auckland.
Tel. 89-2244.

Also by John Stirling
On Four Legs and Two (Benton-Guy)

ISBN 0-86470-006-7

Computersetting by **Newsbrief Publishing**
Design by **Benton-Guy Publishing Ltd**
Illustrations by **Bob Darroch**

Contents

Foreword

This partial autobiography covers the first quarter of a century I spent in New Zealand from 1947. However, for explanation and continuity I have strayed beyond this time.

Where sensitivities may have been involved I have occasionally changed names or omitted them altogether.

It may well be that I have left a few sacred cows needing the vet, but the gibes are usually gentle and a story such as this without comment or opinion would be poor stuff indeed.

I am also grateful to Mrs Rayma Ritchie of Ohaeawai who supplied much of the historical data. My thanks to Bob Darroch for the drawings in this book, including the cover.

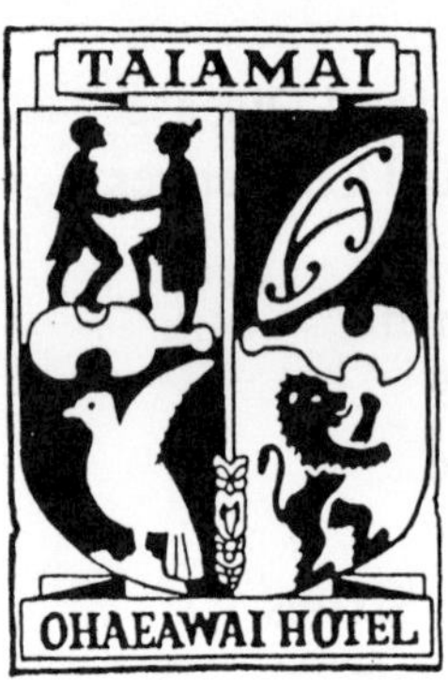

This inn sign, which still swings on its bracket outside the Ohaeawai hotel, tells how the Maori and Pakeha live in friendship near the spot where one of the bloodiest battles of the Maori wars was fought.

It shows the mythical bird perched on the rock from which the district takes its name. It also depicts Maori weapons, implements and playthings, and informs thirsty travellers what beer is on tap.

It was designed by Jim Yearbury of Russell.

Taiamai

Ohaeawai, the village in the Bay of Islands where I lived and worked for nearly 30 years, was only so-called from 1895. Its name, together with the publican's license, was inherited from the original settlement of Ngawha, a few miles to the west.

In pre-European times the district known as Taiamai was well populated with a people who produced kumara and other things from the rich, if sometimes stony volcanic soil. Legend has it that a very large and beautiful white bird — looking something like a pigeon — often settled on a large volcanic rock, preening itself and drinking rainwater from a depression on the summit.

Chief Kaitara and his people marvelled at the size and beauty of the bird and gave it the name Taiamai, which means 'borne inland from the sea.' A rahui or tapu was placed on it for its protection. However, an enemy anxious to decrease the mana or prestige of the protecting chief planned to capture the bird. Legend has it that the bird, sensitive to the ways of man, disappeared and melted into the rock. Later a dying chief, anxious to again see the rock on which the strange bird had rested, visited the place and on his death his spirit also passed into the stone.

The rock, named Te Tino o Taiamai, became an enchanted stone. Maoris passing by often respectfully placed a twig or bunch of greenery at its base. It was believed that such reverence was a protection against evil and also ensured good weather for the traveller.

It stands quite near to the present township of Ohaeawai.

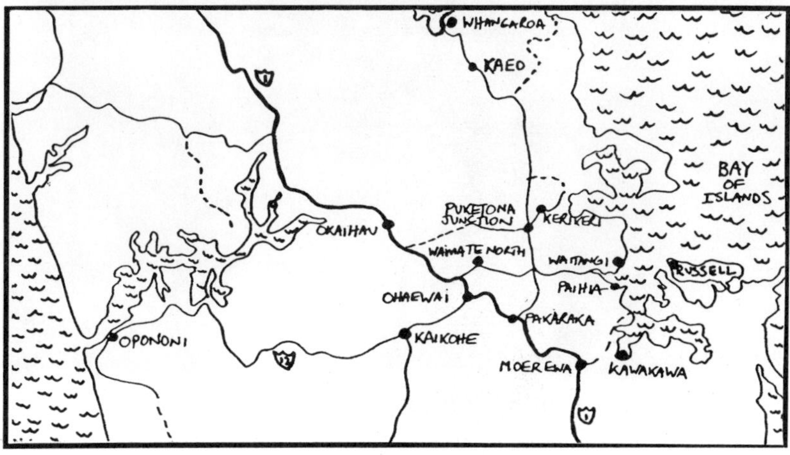

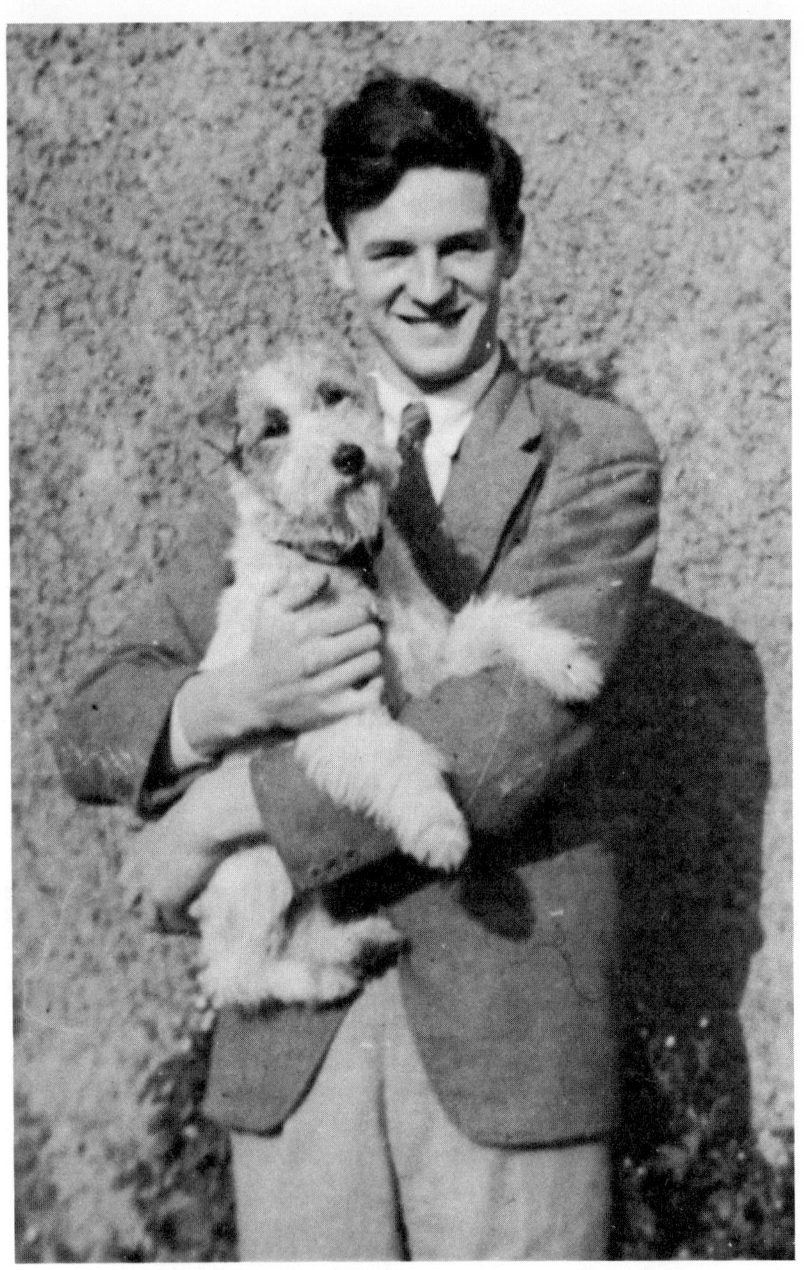

John Stirling as a veterinary student, 1943.

Voyage of Discovery

There is a Happy Land
Far, far away.'
or so I hoped.

My story, like many others, begins on London's River Thames. The time, October 29 1947. The place, the Royal Albert Dock. The vessel, Shaw Savill's *Waiwera* on her eighth voyage to Auckland, New Zealand. Myself, with five years of veterinary school and appetite whetted by three years of war, seeking adventure and maybe reward in a hemisphere to which my previous journeys had not led me.

I had travelled by train from Glasgow the day before through a Britain still rather gloomy and grimy, not yet on the recovery road from the physical and mental impact of war. In London I had said farewell to my father with a tear in my eye and a lump in my throat. It was somewhat softened by a promise that he would join me in a place far away provided the natives were friendly and the roots, which many Scots seem to carry in their suitcase, could be persuaded to establish themselves in another place.

It was by no means easy to secure passage to New Zealand in the late forties with a significant percentage of the world's merchant fleet now resting on the bottom of the sea. Returning servicemen and women, many with spouses acquired while on the business of war, were naturally anxious to return to their native land. Businessmen, keen to establish new contracts where war had destroyed the old, were prominent on the list of passengers. Some, like myself, whose skills were perceived to be needed, were accorded a degree of priority. There were few aboard, so they said, whose journey was not really necessary.

Accommodation on the *Waiwera* had been expanded to meet demand and in many cases husbands and wives had to temporarily forego their conjugal rights as unisex cabins were best for maximising carrying capacity. Attempts to re-establish rights sometimes led to embarrassing discoveries in places such as lifeboats — an appropriate name in more ways than one!

Under a gray sky and a matching river the *Waiwera* was nudged by her tugs into the Thames with her prow pointing east, but soon to turn west. Slowly we began moving through the gathering mist of late afternoon on the first stage of our voyage to the other end of the earth.

By next morning the White Cliffs had been left behind to starboard and the first of the Atlantic rollers were causing a few faces to acquire a greenish tinge and a few chairs to remain vacant at the first breakfast. While many accept this *mal-de-mer* with amusing tolerance, for those badly affected it can be a trying experience. I recall one young lady, a nurse by profession, who was rarely able or willing to stir from her bunk during the whole five weeks of the voyage and arrived at her destination worn out and disillusioned. What the conditions must have been like in years gone by for those afflicted among the sturdy pioneers, whose sailing ships took months to reach their goal, can only be imagined.

Captain Forbes-Moffat and his officers were well aware of the problems which could arise when a lot of people were thrown together in a confined space for quite a long time. Chief Officer Wynyard was soon on deck organising a programme of sports and entertainment which, hopefully, would keep everyone happy and content during the long voyage. Among other things, a passenger's committee was formed to plan and liaise; this was under the chairmanship of General Sir Andrew Thorne, our most distinguished passenger, who, with Lady Thorne, was on his way to visit family and do business in New Zealand.

I had met General Thorne before when, as G.O.C., Scottish Command, he had inspected a guard of honour in Edinburgh. This was composed of members of the student's Home Guard in which I was a lowly private, ready to do battle with any Germans ill-advised enough to make a landing on the soil of Scotland from sea or air. General Thorne could not recollect his former association with his new committee member, but with the gap in our ranks being very considerable at that time, this was no surprise.

For most, seasickness happily disappeared and sea legs were established. Deck tennis, quoits and golf filled the sunlit days. The weather became warmer and shorts and singlets replaced jerseys and slacks.

As is customary at sea, there is always a good deal of anticipatory excitement as the time approaches for a visit to a port of call. Curacao was first on our list. We were to take on fuel oil produced in nearby Venezuela and refined in Curacao itself. Curacao was a small island devoid of vegetation and smelling of oil, the one reason for its habitation.

Willemstad, which looked like a bit of Holland transplanted — and indeed the orange tiles on most of its roofs had come over as ballast on sailing ships — was a welcome break ashore and offered a wide selection of goods, mostly of American origin and seldom seen in Britain for a number of years. The narrow streets were packed with large American cars with little room to manoeuvre. Where they journeyed to and from on such a small island I found hard to imagine.

Unfortunately, the pound sterling, so long the bulwark of the western financial system, was now viewed with a degree of contempt and only those lucky enough to have some American dollars were able to sample the goods and services on offer. The ship did not stay long in any case and we were soon at sea once again. A radio message was received ordering a diversion to Jamaica, where apparently a cargo of grapefruit destined for New Zealand awaited collection.

This was something of a bonus and we were soon to enjoy the hospitality of the local club in Kingston which dispensed, among other things, the traditional rum-based Planter's Punch, a concoction served in long, frosted glasses cooled by ice cubes and surmounted by a variety of tropical fruits, some afloat and others impaled on toothpicks. It was a welcome change from my daily Bass, served by barman Danny during the limited hours he operated. Sipping a Planter's Punch on a balcony overlooking a turquoise bay framed in hibiscus and bougainvillea run riot, a background of cloudless blue interrupted only by the silhouette of palms apparently dancing to some distant calypso, must be close to one of the highest points of man's contentment.

The pound was still thought worthwhile in Kingston, so some touring and shopping was possible. I was even able to afford a typewriter of American origin. It was a machine which stood me in good stead for many years. I discovered though, that the natives were not always friendly. As I penned a postcard in the main post office, my camera which I acquired during war service in Germany, silently and swiftly disappeared from my side.

But, 'pleasures are,' as Burns pointed out 'like snowflakes on a river; a moment there, then gone forever.' And so it was that with most of her complement asleep, dreaming perhaps of a tropical paradise lately visited, the *Waiwera* cast off her links with the land and moved gently into the Caribbean on a course ever further to the south.

After languid Jamaica, Panama was all purpose and industry. There was time for brief visits to Colon and Panama, the terminals at either end of the canal itself, but alas the 'greenback' was needed here more than ever, and this curbed the enthusiasm of many.

The Panama Canal is a most remarkable engineering feat — one of the world's true wonders. The effort, skill and resolution needed to cut a highway of water through which some of the world's largest vessels would pass, was awesome. Carved through a hostile and disease-ridden land it required technical genius to create a system of locks to overcome the problems of varying water levels in two of the world's greatest oceans and the lakes in between.

The passengers of the *Waiwera* were certainly impressed as they watched with awe the massive gates on the locks open and close at the touch of an unseen hand. The busy 'mules' moved smoothly along their tracks shifting our vessel, as effortlessly as a small boy would a toy boat in his bath, a few more yards at a time towards Auckland, New Zealand.

As we moved from the Gulf of Panama, the wind off the Andes was surprisingly cool. Sweaters were again in vogue. However, the Equator was not too far away and the passengers' committee had the task of organising the ceremonies associated with the traditional crossing of the line. We had to plan all sorts of indignities to be perpetrated on those, myself included, who had not passed that way before.

A large and blunt razor of wood was unearthed and quantities of lather prepared. This must have had some secret formula because I had never seen a lather with a personality before. This brew bubbled and frothed like some tub of animated cotton wool. On the day everything went off as planned, the indefatigable Neptune arrived from the deep over the starboard rail aft and proceeded to deal out stiff sentences to all who came to his notice. As the sun moved towards its meeting with the horizon, the bedraggled and often waterlogged graduates were presented with their certificates of achievement. Then, for the most part, they retired to the bar to celebrate and drown the sorrows still afloat after the indignity of the Neptunian tortures.

I know of no more relaxing interlude than leaning on the rail of a boat towards eventide, glass in hand, as a tropical day draws to its close; the sun saying farewell to the day it created as it sinks into the western sea in a display of golds, blues, greens and pinks, reflected perhaps on some misplaced cloud of the darkest blue.

As I absorbed such a scene, and took in the symmetrical pattern of the ship's wake marching in endless tranquil lines to nowhere, I reflected on where I was headed. It was a strangely comforting experience of almost hypnotic character. I had been told that Waiwera, the name of my erstwhile home, meant 'hot water'. I hoped that that would not prove prophetic in respect of my time to come!

Through an advertisement in the *Veterinary Record*, the official professional magazine, I had discovered that New Zealand was in some need of veterinary surgeons. A brother officer in Bangalore, South India, where I had been stationed for a while in 1945, had shown it to me. New Zealand, being one of the world's faraway places, had appeal and challenge. Still restless from the experiences of wartime, I made a provisional application for an appointment to New Zealand under what was called the Veterinary Club system. Here was an important difference from how the profession was organised in the U.K. and in most other places.

In Britain the practices were often large and long-established and run as private concerns. The principal employed assistants, who for the most part aspired to succeeding their bosses one day, or at least acquired a more modest practice of their own.

The New Zealand Club system was organised and controlled by committees of farmers representing the clients of the practice. For convenience, the controlling group was often part of, or closely associated with, a dairy company whose primary function was to handle and market the milk or cream of its farmer members.

While serving with the British Army of the Rhine in Germany I confirmed my previous application to work in New Zealand. During leave in February 1947, I presented myself for an interview with the Agricultural Advisor to the High Commissioner. I went along to his London offices in the Strand, armed with references from my professors in Edinburgh, the Army and a few others. All this must have made some impression, or else the country was simply short of vets. I soon heard that I had the job. As soon as the Army could dispense with my services I would be on my way. My release from the Army came in October 1947 and within a few weeks I was on the high seas.

We steamed through tropic seas with only the company of dolphins and the flying fish fleeing like streaks of silver from the massive bow bisecting the waves.

It is surprising how close-knit a community can become when circumstances throw its members together, even for a comparatively short time. There were a few niggles, but not too many, and the mood became more anticipatory as the weather once again became more temperate. By now it was approaching summer in the southern hemisphere.

Kiwis, the human kind, were quick to point out the increasing brilliance of the Southern Cross at night, set in a sky of dark blue velvet. It was a sure sign for them that they would soon be home.

The second day in December was time for *Dinner Adieu*, the ship's final major effort on her passengers' behalf. A special menu was followed by a dance, with music provided by a gramophone amplified by loudspeakers. These had been hidden by coloured bunting, strung for the occasion between any convenient superstructure offering an anchorage. Dancing on a heaving deck called for a special technique, even though sea legs were by now well and truly established. One second there was an impression of floating on air, the next felt as if the femur was being driven through the pelvic girdle by some devilish force from below. It was nearly time to say goodbye and bring to an end a number of brief but warm friendships, some of which would endure. For me there was even a hint of romance, albeit of a transitory nature, but I guess that would be another story.

We glided through the Hauraki Gulf, identifying and admiring its various islands as they slid by, ever-green and ever-beautiful in the summer sun. Soon the curious green and red roofs of the city's houses were visible. Auckland was clearly no New York or San Francisco. Four stories seemed the limit, and when viewed through binoculars the buildings seemed solid and functional, with their feet on the ground rather than reaching for the sky.

A stock inspector from the Department of Agriculture came aboard when the ship tied up at Princes Wharf and gave me instructions as to my future direction. It appeared I had to report to a place called Hawera in a district called Taranaki, places I had difficulty in pronouncing, far less spelling. A train journey would be involved but connecting services did not dovetail for a couple of days, so meantime I should make the best of things in Auckland.

Left to my own devices, I organised the transfer of my considerable luggage to the railway station from the wharf after a smooth passage through customs. Suitcase in hand I took a taxi to the Star Hotel in Albert Street where I had reserved a room by telegraph while still at sea.

'Well mate,' said my driver, 'and what do you think about New Zealand?'

I explained that I had only been about fifty minutes in the country and comment at that point might be a little premature. He seemed a bit disappointed and tried another tack.

'Wotcha goin' to do now you are here then?'

I explained that I was a vet and hoped to practise my profession.

'Not too many of them around here,' he said. 'What they goin' to pay?'

I indicated that the figure was a little over £600 per annum. He tut-tutted.

'No good mate. I make twice that. I'd give it away. You could do pretty well on the wharves here. If you like I'll give you the phone number of a cobber of mine who's the secretary or something of the wharfies' union and he'll fix you up on Monday.'

I thanked him for his advice and explained that I had a contract and it might not be good public relations to break it within a few days of arrival.

'No sweat there,' he replied. 'They do it all the time; I'll give you this joker's number anyhow.'

By now we had arrived outside the wrought iron facade of the Star Hotel. My taximan wrote a telephone number on the back of a packet lately filled with cigarette tobacco and handed it to me in exchange for his fare. I thanked him for his helpfulness and checked in at reception.

The taximan's advice might not have been all that bad, although I doubt if working on the wharves was quite my cup of tea. At the time of my arrival only a handful of vets practised in Auckland and they were mainly associated with the major racing clubs. The small animal population, which even then must have been considerable, was largely unserviced in a veterinary sense — a land of opportunity indeed and in hindsight an opportunity missed, but hindsight is of course always the easiest of options.

I must say that the Star Hotel had a style and character which impressed me and continued to do so for many years. My family and I would often stay there in the years to come. Morning tea was served with a silver teaspoon and monogrammed china accompanied by the *New Zealand Herald* and two biscuits within a few minutes either side of seven o'clock — such a nice way to start the day. There was time to reflect before committing oneself to anything. I was surprised to see in the *Herald* that my name was mentioned as a passenger off the *Waiwera*. I was suitably impressed, but noted that I warranted only a couple of lines, whereas General Thorne got half a column.

The Star's dining room was also impressive with its tables set at different levels and heavy with starched linen. The menu was supported by side services bearing all manner of delicacies. After the constraints of a severely rationed Britain, the food was an absolute delight. There was bacon with two eggs, and porridge with cream which could only be coaxed from its jug with difficulty.

The dining room was presided over by a lady in a tight-fitting black dress who effortlessly administered her charge with Sergeant-Major-like precision.

Dinner was at 6.15 and that meant what it said — no nonsense like 6.30 or 6.45. If you missed, you missed, for other hotels kept to a tight schedule. Restaurants were largely unheard of and the many licensed premises closed right on six with the patrons happily spilling on to the streets to pursue their uncertain way home perhaps to meet, like Tam O'Shanter, their dame, 'Gathering her brows like a gath'rin' storm — nursing her wrath to keep it warm.'

For the first time in my life, and most likely the last, I felt homesick. Sheer distance from my native heath plus the sudden loss of friends, contributed to this. As I had already spent a number of years away from home, some in foreign places, the symptoms rather surprised me. I had no relations at all in New Zealand and clearly my choice was to be a self-made man or no man at all. The options were few!

I had no intention of nursing my sorrows in a hotel bedroom, so I decided to attend the evening performance in the Civic Theatre in Queen Street. I had always been a keen cinema fan and if anything could dispel homesickness surely this was it. The programme was presented in a manner almost identical to the northern hemisphere — down to the organ rising from the depths in front of the stage to provide entertainment between screenings while patrons arrived and departed, purchased ice creams and confections and did all the other things that people do in cinemas at such times.

It was here that I made my first New Zealand *faux pas*. At that time I was like most of my generation, a fairly heavy smoker and when I had settled in

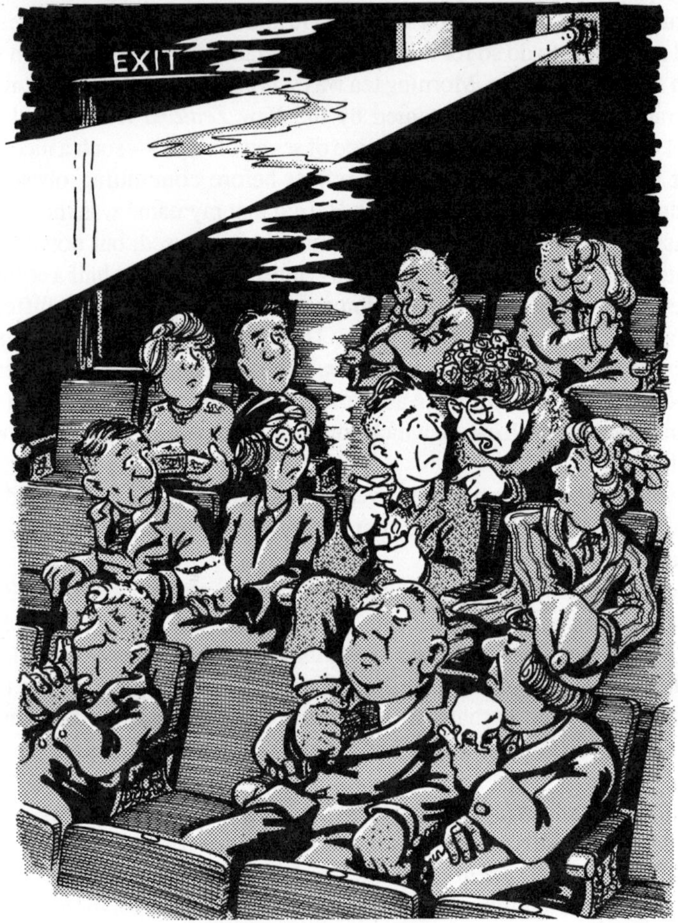

my seat it was not long before I felt the need to light up a 'State Express' from one of the duty free tins I had purchased on the *Waiwera*. I blew a cloud of blue smoke into the air above and was rewarded by a tap on the shoulder from a lady seated behind.

In a peppermint scented whisper to my left ear she advised me, 'Excuse me, young man, but in cinemas smoking is not allowed. Please put out your

16

cigarette or I will call the manager.'

This was all news to me nevertheless but an instruction not to be ignored. I hastily complied with the request. I had no wish to be returned to the footpath before the programme had even started.

On later reflection I scored this as a plus for New Zealand. In Britain where smoking in cinemas was permitted it was sometimes difficult to identify the characters on the screen through the thick tobacco haze which usually prevailed. Although ash trays were provided one was extremely lucky to preserve one's clothes from scorching or worse from the showers of hot ash often deposited at random from contiguous smokers.

Next morning while still in bed enjoying my tea and biscuits, the phone rang by the bedside. Stuart Findlay, a fellow voyager from the *Waiwera* and I believed, a businessman of some prominence in the city, enquired if I would like to attend a race meeting with him and his family at Avondale. I later discovered that he was a member of the committee. I readily agreed as I had nothing else planned. Soon after breakfast Stuart's son picked me up in his Peugeot car and we quickly arrived at Avondale with the first race about to start.

I had had quite a lot to do with horses during my war service and was interested to have this early experience in New Zealand. It was clear that racing was a major attraction in the country with a large crowd present, seemingly all intent upon picking the winners of the day. The horses looked fit and performed well, although I thought their grooming left a bit to be desired. Perhaps the shortage of labour in New Zealand compared with, for instance, India and Germany — countries I had lately visited, had something to do with this.

It was a happy day if a bit exhausting, explaining to the many people to whom I was introduced why I was here and where my future lay. The first question was easier to answer than the second! I even backed a winner, although I must confess, with the benefit of inside information.

Taranaki Bound — Locum Tenens

In the late afternoon of the next day it was time to resume my travels with this place Hawera my target. It sounded almost as far away as China and anybody I spoke to in Auckland about it seemed to confirm that impression. I reassembled my luggage and boarded a train with New Plymouth the immediate destination — that was at least a lot easier to pronounce. A fair cross section of the youth of Auckland seemed to be on the platform seeing somebody off, and their song and dance was uplifting to a still rather lonely immigrant from far away.

The stimulus did not persist however. The train, as it swayed its way through the gathering dusk and pastures of South Auckland and the Waikato, brought back memories of a similar journey I made in India from Lahore to Madras. Both compared comfort-wise but there were some differences. Here it was not necessary to keep the door locked to exclude non fare-paying passengers and, as far as I could see, nobody was carried on the roof.

After a couple of hours or so it was dark and we arrived at a place called Frankton. There was a lot of jostling, distribution of pillows and rugs, soft drinks and, above all, tea and pies before we set off into the night in what I presumed was a westerly direction.

The train rumbled on through the night, stopping often for reasons I did not know, although on one occasion a passing official in response to a bleary-eyed enquiry, said that cattle were on the line somewhere and had to be chased off. Arrival time at New Plymouth was 5 a.m. and the place seemed to be totally uninhabited. I was not due to leave again until nine, so I managed to organise some breakfast in a nearby boarding house whose still sleepy management seemed a bit surprised by the request. At that time New Plymouth was not the energy centre of New Zealand it is today, but mainly a service town for the dairy industry. At the time I arrived I guess most farmers were still in their cowsheds and hence the 'deserted village' atmosphere.

My next conveyance was the *Taranaki Flyer*, a misnomer as it turned out, for the journey south was punctuated by frequent halts, some of which looked like private railway stations. The merchandise transported was as interesting to me as it was varied. Coils of wire, cans of milk or cream, crates of beer, bundles of plants and even half-a-dozen Jersey calves with only their heads protruding from the sacks secured around their necks designed to prevent their premature escape.

The slow progress on some inclines caused me to wonder if the train was moving at all, but the frequent halts gave me my first opportunity to observe rural New Zealand. It would have been a traveller of poor response who failed to be impressed. The fields — I had yet to learn to call them paddocks — flowed westwards like some gently undulating magic carpet. Green and symmetrical, they were divided by fences of wire or boxthorn hedge. They flowed towards the crushed green velvet of Egmont's bush-clad foothills stretching ever upwards toward that spectacular and still snow-capped volcanic peak of perfect proportion. Egmont presided over all with a majesty I could only regard with awe as it glistened in the summer sun.

Of equal interest to me was the animal population and it was clear that at least in this part of the country the Jersey cow was queen. Although it did not register at the time, the Jersey was an animal with which I was to form a close association in the years ahead. There were, of course, some very good reasons why the Jersey should dominate. The climate of most of the country suited the breed admirably, farmers were paid on the amount of cream they produced rather than the volume of milk and the Jersey breed had a higher percentage of cream in the milk than any other. The Jersey cow being one of the smaller members of her species, could live in bigger numbers on fewer acres and was generally of a quiet disposition. But later I was to encounter a few who did prove to be aggressive and ill-mannered.

And so my train of slow speed and few passengers proceeded across the sunlit land and late afternoon pulled into the station at Hawera near the southern coast of the bulge which is Taranaki. I observed a burly figure in khaki shorts and a short-sleeved pullover, accompanied by an interesting looking red setter with lolling tongue, expectantly casting their eyes in my direction. This was Jack Stewart, even then a well-known pillar of the profession in New Zealand, and later to grace some of its high offices.

Jack was clearly glad to see me and soon had my considerable luggage stowed in the back of his blue V-8 car with Mick the dog and a miscellaneous collection of veterinary equipment, most of which was familiar. Board had been arranged for me with a Mrs Rowlands of Disraeli Street. The idea was that being a new chum to New Zealand I should spend some time with Jack before going on elsewhere. In this way it was hoped that the rough edges would be knocked off before being exposed to my ultimate clients who might otherwise have been less than impressed by a rookie vet from the other side of the world trying to teach them their business. I soon discovered that the technique of knocking off rough edges was very much a matter of being thrown in at the deep end.

Jack had a number of meetings to attend in Wellington and other places plus a wedding in Auckland before Christmas, now fast approaching. Any vet was better than no vet, and he had to take advantage of the opportunity my arrival presented. The time available for tuition and induction was thus limited and it was not long before I was sole charge in quite a large and varied practice. Fortunately, the calving of cows in New Zealand is made to coincide with the spring flush of grass, apart from in the town milk industry. Luckily for me by the time I reached Hawera the cows had as they say, dropped their bundles and overcome or succumbed to the numerous problems of early lactation.

Number 10 Disraeli Street was an old wooden house with quite a large number of rooms. The widowed landlady took about half-a-dozen boarders, mostly young people working in town. There was a stock agent, an insurance broker, a hairdresser and a couple of typists, the latter three being female. I think my fellow boarders sensed a difference, although to be fair they did not exploit it. Some of my luggage bore the legend 'Major J. Stirling', a relic of my army days. I think the stock agent found this a bit hard to take as he had recently been discharged from the New Zealand Army with the rank of Lance Corporal. He most likely felt I should have been in an officers' mess somewhere and not in his boarding house in Disraeli Street.

However I had read that New Zealand was an egalitarian country, so I guess it cut both ways. It was a refreshing contrast to the snobbery and class distinction, a legacy of Victorian times, which still lingered in Britain between the wars. But as Sir Keith Holyoake described it, 'Here we are all equal — but some are more equal than others.' In New Zealand to this day, the lower echelons are often suspicious of the higher, while the latter view their less fortunate brothers with a degree of condescension so subtle that it is not always recognised even by those who bestow it.

It was finally time to go back to work. I made a few calls with Jack but mostly I worked on my own, applying first principles and consulting with my erstwhile boss when he was around. It was not an easy time, for although I had acquired a good collection of excellent veterinary instruments in Hamburg at bargain prices — they were ex-Wehrmacht — I didn't feel it worthwhile to unpack them in a temporary situation. The drugs available were not always known to me, the pattern of stock disease different and the clients, as clients do, always appeared to feel vaguely let down when a new assistant and not the boss responded to their call.

One case I attended still stands out in my memory. I received a message from the office of a local accountant who doubled as secretary of the Veterinary Club and the local racing club. He explained that a horse at the Alexander stud at Maxwell 30 miles away was in a bad way and needed Jack Stewart pronto. As Jack Stewart was arguing some case in Wellington this looked like one for the locum, so I revved up the old truck and set off at a good clip down the highway leading south.

I arrived in just a bit over half-an-hour obviously impressing the horse's owner by the speed of my arrival, if not by the fact that it was I and not Jack Stewart who had appeared. The surroundings and the owner appeared affluent and this was further borne out when I was told that Coronach, for that was the name of the animal, was a stallion imported from Britain and was one of New Zealand's better-known and most successful sires.

Coronach, an impressive chestnut stallion, was in a loose box in which he moved around restlessly. He stopped only to give me a worried look before throwing himself to the ground with a groan and a grunt, then stretching himself out, extending his neck and panting. He was clearly not at all happy.

I asked all the usual questions and learned among other things that the day before, Coronach had managed to open the door of a shed where fodder was stored and imbibed rather more of his usual ration than was obviously good for him. This latter piece of information was useful to me as it indicated that the horse could be suffering from uncomplicated spasmodic colic, an equine indigestion often associated with a feeding binge. It was rather like the stomach ache of a small boy, having over-indulged at a party.

'I think colic is the trouble,' was my tentative diagnosis.

'I know that,' was the terse reply, ' but what do we do?'

Now, although the owner probably didn't appreciate the fact, I had had quite a lot of experience with horses and their problems in the British Army. I had served under the watchful eye of older, often Irish, senior officers in the Royal Army Veterinary Corps, who I believe were the best equine diagnosticians in certain fields the world has yet produced. I had long ago formed the conclusion that colic was either of a simple type which recovered with or without treatment, or a serious type which proved fatal whether treatment was applied or not. The simple type, which I hoped I was dealing with, usually passed off in a few hours and all I normally prescribed in the army was to have the patient gently led round in circles. This prevented self-injury caused by throwing himself violently to the ground or against a nearby hazard. It also prevented the hundred-odd feet of intestines from twisting in a tangle which always proved fatal. Another serious and often fatal form of colic was impaction where the intestines became blocked by a food mass.

There was something about the state of Coronach I did not like and which kept ringing the alarm bells which the experienced human and animal physician often hear for no particular reason. The pain was too continuous, while in ordinary colic it was usually intermittent. The pulse was faster than it should have been and the membrane of the eye was a dirty red instead of a salmon pink.

I asked the owner to bring his horse out into the yard and apply a hobble to the near hind leg. This would give me personal protection while I carried out a rectal examination. To lubricate the arm I requested a bucket of warm water and some soap, the usual prepared lubricant not for the time being available from my repertoire of medicines. The owner complied, although he clearly thought that I should be getting on with the cure and not fiddling about with hobbles and buckets of soapy water.

It is possible to palpate most of the contents of the abdominal contents in horses and cattle through the wall of the rectum as it is a passage commodious enough to admit the hand and arm of the operator. As I introduced my well-lubricated arm — in those days there were no refinements like protective gloves — Coronach tensed and was only prevented from throwing himself to the ground by the timely intervention of his owner jerking his halter and slapping his flank.

I thought that I could detect a firm enlargement in the intestinal wall almost out of reach; it could have been an impaction but it was indefinite and not so clear as to be a basis for prognosis.

'All I can suggest,' I concluded, 'is that you keep him on his feet and walk him around in circles. I'll give him a sedative by injection to ease the pain.'

'Is that all you can do?' enquired the owner, clearly of the opinion that he wasn't getting value for his money.

'I'm afraid so,' I replied. 'Any purgative or the like might only aggravate the condition and would certainly cause a lot more pain. He is showing some symptoms of what could be a twist or impaction and these are serious conditions.'

On this unsatisfactory note I left. Jack Stewart told me next day that the owner had rung him in his Wellington hotel the night before and he had called in to see Coronach on his way home. All was apparently well, although the owner and his family had had a long night attending their charge.

Although recovery was apparently complete on this occasion it was no surprise to me when I read in the newspaper about a year later that the well known sire Coronach had succumbed to an attack of colic. My apprehension, I felt, had been justified, and my one regret was that I was not then in a position to carry out a post mortem which might have revealed a long-standing stricture or blockage which eventually had led to the fatal abdominal catastrophe.

My memoirs at this time would not be complete without reference to the vehicle with which I had been provided. This was a pre-war V-8 truck whose powerful engine drove it along the well-surfaced and mostly straight roads of South Taranaki at a good rate. The brakes were not all that reliable and some loose springs had penetrated the leather upholstery, creating a potential hazard for driver and passenger alike. This had been minimised by some old folded fertiliser sacks strategically placed but which required continual readjustment.

The attendant at the garage which had long serviced the aging vehicle told me that the chassis, most likely as a result of some accident, had a significant bend. This explained why it was necessary to keep a very firm compensatory grip on the steering wheel to stop the vehicle veering to the left and heading into a ditch or tree.

On one occasion when I returned to town from the country the streets were filled with excited people. I thought that the Russians must have moved into Germany or somewhere.

'Did you feel the shake?' enquired the attendant when I stopped at the garage for petrol.

'She was a real beaut; knocked the oil cans off the shelf in there and stopped the petrol pumps for a while.'

I was sorry to have missed my first earthquake. Apparently the vibrations generated by the old truck were higher on the Richter scale than those of a mere earthquake.

As the days passed into weeks I became increasingly more restless, although the environment in which I found myself was pleasant enough. However, I wanted to relocate and, as they say, do my own thing. There was another reason. About this time I had the very great fortune to meet the lady who was to be my wife. Wedding plans were discussed but the where and the when were as yet unclear.

Mere human wishes, however determined or impatient, were not enough to overcome the great New Zealand inertia surrounding the Christmas festival. Decisions were not made, except perhaps on the cricket field or tennis court. Moves, unless from home to beach or for strictly social reasons, were difficult to organise in a practical sense. In late January the country gave a final yawn and, among other things, I was told my destination was to be the Bay of Islands. Hasty reference to the map showed that the place was quite a long way away, partly over paths I had already crossed. The name sounded attractive enough — even romantic and intriguing — but what was the reality? Official detail was sketchy and appeared a bit defensive.

Phrases like, 'If you don't like it maybe in about a year we'll find you a better possie' were bandied about. The locals had little knowledge and less interest in anything north of Auckland and the only information I could gather was in a farming sense and maybe in other ways, it was 'patchy'. What that meant I had yet to discover.

Go North Young Man

And so it came to pass that early February I was on the road once again. I did not know whether the *Taranaki Flyer* flew in both directions but in the interests of speed, change of scenery and possibly of comfort, I persuaded a local farmer who was heading south with a load of pigs for market to deliver myself and my luggage to Palmerston North. From there the main trunk line proceeded across awesome chasms with rushing torrents racing towards the faraway sea. The skill of those who had built this railway and its bridges, no doubt with minimal equipment, left me in wonder. The mountains, although their coating of snow was less than in winter, reminded me of the Himalayas, although less crowded and therefore more pleasing to the eye.

There was another diversion of a different sort. I shared a compartment with a talkative Irishman who had lived in New Zealand for many years. Like many of his nationality he was fluent of speech and had an enduring love for the horse. When he learned that I was a vet his interest quickened and he gave me some off-the-cuff tuition on the doping of trotting horses. He recounted that it was a skill he had developed to the point where he could stimulate any horse to super-equine performance or, alternatively, tranquillise it so that after a given distance it would languish and allow its heavily backed rival to pass the post first. This was all news to me and maybe some of it was true. Tests now applied randomly to competing race horses were not then in vogue, and some, like my Irish friend, may have taken advantage of this omission.

I reached Auckland early evening and was told that no train would head further north that day so I felt that I could do no better than renew my acquaintance with the Star Hotel. The hotel was as welcoming as ever and, as it turned out, was to be my last experience of relative luxury for some time.

Next morning I was left with the feeling Livingstone or Stanley must have felt. I had been told that I was going where no vet had gone before. Despite my trepidation I returned to the station, assembled my luggage and headed north just 20 minutes later.

Despite the feeling that we were moving backwards, we cleared suburbia with its panorama of backyards, vegetable gardens, washing on the line, and small children on tricycles and moved into the countryside of North Auckland.

Well, I had been told it was 'patchy' and that's what it seemed to be. Some fields were green but there was also a lot of gorse which I recognised and ti-tree which I didn't.

After three hours or so we reached Whangarei where we stopped for tea and pies. It turned out to be a much longer stop than anticipated. A summer deluge had caused a slip which had blocked the line further north and this would need to be cleared before further progress could be made. After another hour the train proceeded through more suburbia and then through the sunlit hills of the north. The flats in many cases were covered in miniature lakes (or should I say lochs?) indicative of heavy rainfall in the not too distant past. We edged cautiously along the side of the slip, now cleared while workmen clad in khaki shorts and blue singlets leaned on shovels and waved us onwards, indicating that all was well.

Late afternoon the train halted at Otiria Junction. My destination proved to be an undistinguished looking collection of shacks, sheds and sidings. Nearby cattle yards and a building with a much-carved facade, later identified as a Maori meeting house, provided variety. Awaiting my arrival was a short, fair-haired man, older than myself, but still young, with glasses and a Model A Ford car of uncertain vintage. This car was to play a part in my story later but for the moment I accepted the assurance that it was a useful vehicle for traversing flooded paddocks. Its high clearance facilitated the negotiation of rocks often found on farmlands and even the roads in this part of the world.

John Phillips, for this was the name of my new acquaintance, was the secretary of the Bay of Islands and Kaikohe Veterinary Service.

As we passed along the road, twin plumes of dust from the Model A added still another coating to the tall grass and shrubbery of the wayside. John Phillips mentioned that it had been decided I should be located at a place called Ohaeawai, which apparently was the geographic centre of my practice. Board had been arranged with one Eric Baldwin, whose brother Chappie was a prominent director of the Bay Dairy Company which was under the chairmanship of Syd Smith, the local M.P. I suspected that Syd Smith, who was later to become an Under-Secretary for Agriculture, may have used his influence in Wellington to secure my appointment. Hens' teeth and vets had much in common numerically and new appointees were widely canvassed.

We soon turned off the Otiria Road onto State Highway 1 and proceeded some way along a bitumen-sealed road. The seal gave me some misplaced encouragement as it soon turned out that Kaikohe's main street and a few yards through some of the townships, were the only lengths of sealed road in my entire practice.

Tea and cakes with John and his wife Myra was followed by a preliminary discussion in the Bay Dairy Company office, a brick building that was a bit ahead of its time. It was decided that we should pay a courtesy call on 'Sec' Martin, the newly-elected chairman of the veterinary committee. Sec was a farmer of forthright manner who once told me that if he was guided by his conscience, he would sell his farm and give the money to the starving Chinese — brave words indeed! By the time we arrived at Sec's place he was milking. Preliminary introductions over, he at once showed me a lame cow about which he sought advice — I promised attention if not necessarily cure when I had the necessary medicines.

As the shadows were beginning to lengthen John and I headed north along Highway 1, and quarter-of-an-hour later the Model A was chugging its way up the last dusty incline to Ohaeawai, my destination. The township was set in country which had clearly been the centre of significant volcanic activity. As we completed the last stage of our journey I could identify at least two volcanic cones silhouetted against the setting sun to the west and north. Yet another larger peak was floodlit by the same sun to the south. Some paddocks had been cleared of stone and tidily and effectively built into dry stone walls, such as I had seen in Yorkshire and parts of Scotland. But in many others the boulders remained where they had fallen, propelled with the violence of eruption from their parent volcanoes long ago.

The day was drawing to a close and John was anxious to return home as he knew that the lights on his car were not reliable. He suggested that I spend the night at the local hotel and said that next morning he would call and continue my introduction to more people and places.

The wooden Ohaeawai Hotel looked as if its main function was the dispensing of the products of the country's two main breweries to an eager clientele. For a while I joined the system and as I pondered a tankard of ale before dinner I felt that the long day had been one of achievement and even fulfilment. At least I had arrived, even if I could see a few problems ahead.

In Britain, a new graduate (because in the bovine sense that is what I was) was carefully cosseted on entry to a new practice by principals and senior staff and his approach and techniques carefully monitored. After all, the practice was an important and very personal institution whose good name a newcomer could in no circumstances be allowed to prejudice. After a period of working under direct supervision a few 'easy' cases might be tackled by the newcomer and in a year or two he might achieve acceptance by clients and near equality by colleagues. In my case none of this was going to happen. My knowledge of cattle practice, clearly my *raison d'etre*, was fairly standard for a new British graduate but maybe not all that comprehensive. It was going to be applied in a land as far away as possible from where it had been acquired and with a clientele which had no clear idea of what a vet was supposed to do.

In these early times farmers used to inquire if I calved cows or 'blew up a bag' — the term given to the sometimes effective but now outdated treatment for milk fever of inflating the udder with a bicycle pump. My nearest professional colleagues in practice were located at Warkworth and Ruawai, more than 100 miles away. From a practical point of view this was as near as the moon; relief or consultation was not going to be easy. I was sure that a massive education and public relations effort lay ahead of me and this proved to be so. However, at the end of the first day I was content, already part of the place which was to be my home for many years.

On the Road

The next day John Phillips came early and we were soon on the road — but not for long. The farm where my board had been arranged extended nearly into the township of Ohaeawai itself. Eric Baldwin was a pleasant, spare man of helpful disposition and ready smile. He milked 80 cows on his own — quite a big herd for that time. He was a man handy with saw and pipe wrench whose industry was reflected not only in the hay barn and piggery on his farm, but also in community projects such as the school baths. When I finally managed to buy my own house, Eric expertly laid the paths in concret, and practically unassisted he built a substantial bach at Paihia by the sea.

I think that Eric, maybe better than anyone else, understood the dilemma of a new, young vet catapulted from one end of the world to the other into an environment, though not hostile, very much 'wait and see'. Eric was a fountain of knowledge about local farming and people, having lived in the district all his life. His advice was invaluable. I well recall one of my first calls was to a heifer owned by Eric's brother Chappie and considered something of a firebrand. Eric, more as a protector than a spectator, elected to accompany me. Chappie had indicated that he didn't expect much could be done and had his shotgun ready. However he felt he should support the new service. On this unpromising note Eric and I arrived and I inspected the heifer. Soon I had the fractured metatarsus straightened and the ends of the bone held in alignment by half-a-dozen plaster bandages reinforced by some chicken wire. I was obviously showing early signs of Kiwi resourcefulness.

All this had made quite a profound impression on Chappie, enhanced about a month later when I called to remove the bandages, revealing a leg returned to normal in every way. I had acquired a valuable supporter in Chappie who was a great talker, and I have no doubt the case received maximum publicity.

I was allotted a room at the back of the Baldwin house for myself and another much smaller one off the wash-house for my gear. This room was quite inadequate and had little storage space and no water supply, but it had to do. I little thought that in about ten years I would own the house and farm on which I stood and that later my son would sleep in the room I flatteringly called my surgery.

Later in the morning the transport company truck arrived and delivered my luggage from Otiria, and my instruments saw the light of day for the first time since leaving Scotland. I also sent off a list of medicines which I thought I might need to the National Dairy Association in Auckland, the nearest supplier of veterinary equipment. A few further tools of trade were also needed. In those days medicines were not always supplied in the attractive packets, bottles and pottles of today. Medicines like the sulphates of iron and copper, ammonium carbonate, nux vomica, gentian and ginger often had to be pounded from crystal to powder in a substantial mortar using its companion pestle, before combining and dispensing as required. Calcium borogluconate, possibly the most common injection used in bovine practice, had to be prepared by first dissolving the boracic acid powder in boiling water before adding the prescribed amount of calcium gluconate. A mortar and pestle, as well as a one gallon electric urn, was therefore added to my list.

I was soon to experience my first sample of farm fare. Lunch was an example of how New Zealand farmers, no doubt conscious of the large amounts of meat and dairy produce their country exported, did their best to reduce the exportable surplus by consuming large quantities themselves! Steak and kidneys in an appetising stew followed a bowl of nutritious looking soup. I thought we were finished, but not so. Still to come was a generous portion of what looked like plum pudding effectively camouflaged by cream from a large jug obviously designed to hold milk for a large family. Cups of tea and large slabs of chocolate cake followed. I could see that my waistline was one of the things I was going to have to watch most closely!

Time had indeed flown and the weekend was at hand. As I had no medicines I could not yet start work and John Phillips had suggested to me that I might like to accompany him and a friend on a visit to the Bay of Islands. I readily agreed and he picked me up in the Model A, introducing me to his friend — an insurance agent named, as I recall it, Barret. A stop was made at Moerewa to pick up a 'cut lunch' (new word for me) from Johns's home and we were off over the very windy and very dusty road which led to the Bay.

I was un-prepared for the magnificence of the spectacle which greeted us as we moved down the last grade leading to the waterfront, still partially hidden by a magnificent Norfolk Pine. The Bay was blue and beautiful and in those days although it was high summer, only a few picnicked or frolicked in the placid waters of Paihia's beach.

We drove along the waterfront admiring the historic church of stone and roof of slate, towards the wharf where the *Bay Belle* awaited our pleasure. We were ready to proceed on what I was told was the Cream Trip.

Paihia in those days had but a few houses on the waterfront and they were mostly owned by inland farmers who used them only occasionally. There were no motels and the only hotel was a two-storeyed wooden structure in Bayview Road; this was destroyed in a spectacular fire in the 1970's. There was a cinema made up from the union of a number of Nissen hut segments — perhaps relics of wartime. The cinema was owned and operated by a gentleman named Dyke who personally presided over proceedings with an iron hand and an unwavering torch beam. This he unerringly directed at any showing of undue emotion, even if at times it appeared justified by the antics of Clark Gable or perhaps Errol Flynn on the screen out front. Another of Mr Dyke's entrepreneurial activities was to supply milk products to the residents of Paihia and the few visitors who arrived. The milk was produced by a small herd of Jersey cows which used to graze paddocks quite close to the centre of the township. I got to know Mr Dyke quite well later, as from time to time I attended his cows when they needed veterinary attention.

Meantime, we proceeded along the wharf and joined half-a-dozen others and some freight which included cream cans, coils of rope, fishing nets, crayfish pots and a miscellaneous collection of steel pipes and rubber tubing which looked as if it might be part of a milking machine. The *Bay Belle* soon cast off and headed across the harbour to Russell, asleep in the sun. Here some left and others embarked while more freight was loaded and secured.

The Cream Trip, which still survives in name as a tourist attraction, was in those days a multifunctional affair with the cartage of cream an important part of the business. The cream was picked up from a few islands, but more especially from the eastern seaward side of the Russell peninsula. There was then no road access, or if there was it was so primitive as to make the highway of the sea more attractive. Later, it was my lot and my privilege to visit some of these outlandish places, the owners usually picking me up in their boats from either Paihia or Opua. In one case an elderly gentleman with an ailing Labrador, hired a special launch for my transport.

Leaving Russell we headed into a gentle easterly. Noting the tall flagstaff carrying the union flag marking Waitangi across the harbour to port, we soon rounded Tapeka Point accompanied by a shoal of cavorting porpoises chasing their prey between the rocks. Seawards, clouds of birds indicated the presence of shoal fish, at that time present in great numbers.

As we rounded Tapeka the breeze freshened. We proceeded along the Russell peninsula making three stops to drop cream cans and stores, replacing them with full or partly full cans of cream, the product of the morning's and previous evening's milking. In one case a jetty of sorts had been built but in the other two, transfer was by boats, small and of shallow draught. One was propelled by a coughing and spluttering outboard and the other by oars wielded by the muscular arms of the farmer-sailor.

Again a change of course north-east and we headed for Otehei Bay. Here Zane Gray had established his fishing lodge in days gone by, and established many records for the great numbers of shark and billfish he and his friends caught. Perhaps because of my concern about living things I have never been able to identify the pleasure in playing — a strange word in the circumstances — a creature at the end of a line for sometimes many hours before its escape or demise.

At Otehei Bay a stop was made for lunch and some donned swimming gear to take advantage of the incredibly clear and apparently warm water. Scots of my generation did not often enter deep water unless they had to. Shoals of small fish, such as piper and herring, competed with their larger but more clumsy human counterparts.

With the sun still high in the sky and accompanied by a flock of seagulls identifying the unwanted remnants of someone's lunch, we moved gently out of this peaceful haven and into the open bay where the wind blew and the spray flew. Our vessel rose and fell to the swell and one or two passengers looked as if their lunch might not stay with them. There were more porpoises and shoal fish as we headed up the Kerikeri inlet. Here our skipper pointed out Marsden Cross, a notable memorial set on a green hillside overlooking the sea and erected to the memory of Samuel Marsden. Marsden was a missionary and early settler who first arrived there back in 1814 on the brig *Active*. I later discovered that Marsden's name was incorporated in that of a number of early families in the district, who later became my clients. A horseshoe turn saw us again head for Russell and Paihia as the sun started to sink in the west and the shadows lengthened.

It was a remarkable day and although I made many more visits to the Bay of Islands for business or pleasure, this first visit had been particularly special. A less pleasant memento of the day was evident in bed that night with tingling on my nose, neck and back. Within a day or two the redness was replaced by much itchiness and shedding of skin. It was a timely reminder of the strength of the sun in this southern land.

With another week about to start, the carrier truck delivered two very large packing cases filled mostly with veterinary medicines from Auckland. Armed with instruments and now medicines, my assault on the animal population of the Bay of Islands was imminent; but how was I to get to where the animals were?

Just as I was ruminating on this latest problem a farmer arrived at the door and told me he had a cow which was unable to calve and he would take me to her if I would step into his car parked outside. Full of enthusiasm I grabbed some gear and the necessary medicines from amongst the straw packing. As it happened it proved to be an anti-climax. The patient confined in the cowshed, had just delivered a bonny brown Jersey calf with a white star on his forehead. Already it was seeking sustenance on unsteady legs. The mother gave her owner and myself a look of what can only be described as disdain and returned to the more important task of mothering her new offspring. The owner and myself returned from whence we had come.

Such a transport system was clearly not one of permanence. An earlier visit to garages in nearby Kaikohe did not give me a lot of encouragement. New cars were very scarce. As far as I could see only traffic officers, stock agents and the like, seemed favoured with these. No doubt they offered long-term business prospects to the car dealers. Pioneer vets, while viewed with a degree of interest as a new species, did not excite a lot of enthusiasm when the provision of a new vehicle was mentioned. At last there was a glimmer of hope when a dealer told me he had a car which was near-new and could be available. The car was an immediate post-war English model and I bought it for £600.

A word about this car. Cars built in England about this time could not be said to be the best that country had produced in the past and would produce in the future. Mine was no exception. I had been sold something of a pup. I learned later that the car, originally acquired for the use of the dealer's wife, had been disposed of because of an unreliable and temperamental braking system. The brakes required the driver to partially rise from his seat to generate enough muscular power to operate the system. But they were only part of the problem. The frame of the driver's seat, perhaps because of continual pounding on the bumpy roads, soon gave way and left me for a day or two sitting on an orange box while the ailing frame was welded together. My mechanic could only shake his head in disbelief. The original blue paint soon succumbed to the southern sun, mud and rain leaving a whitish, washed-out effect.

However pioneers can't have everything. With medicines and instruments in the boot and back seat and myself in the front, I was ready to go.

The vet's phone started ringing. It didn't stop for more than 20 years.

Patient and Client

In considering a title for this part of the book I wondered whether 'client' or 'patient' should have precedence. In human medicine the two are often synonymous but not so in its veterinary counterpart.

Which should come first was also often something of a problem in the field and occasionally presented a dilemma not too easy to solve. The urgency and even anguish which I, and later perhaps more often my wife sensed over the telephone wires, reflected a justifiable concern on the part of owners for the welfare of their animals. Sometimes mere urgency was replaced by an aggressive trend, reflecting a demand for immediate attention ahead of all others, whatever their need. The veterinary practitioner had to be something of a diplomat in the handling of his client while preserving his primary obligation to his patient. It was not a question of 'first come, first served' but how close to death or how persistent the pain, which counted in my book when establishing where to go first.

I suppose that in more established parts of the world, where a veterinary service of one sort or another had been in place for many years, the passage of time had moulded a facility of communication and understanding which largely sorted these matters out for themselves. Where the institution was new and still novel, the problems of communication and assessment of priority were at best difficult and at worst daunting.

It had been decided that the office of the Bay of Islands Transport Company, centrally situated in the Ohaeawai township, would be a suitable depot where messages relating to the veterinary needs of the district could be recorded for my attention. The lady in charge of the office soon found herself in a new frontline, but to her credit she remained unruffled and wrote down what she heard on the telephone in copperplate longhand. The message, however well written, did not always convey as much as it might have. One from my casebook, for example, 'Taffy Jones — crook cow — go thro' Fergie's place — our culvert washed out' presented something of an exercise in extra sensory perception. It was a new skill I was to develop to a fairly high degree.

Animal owners, in reporting their need for a veterinary presence, varied considerably in their approach. Some had already confidently diagnosed the trouble, a diagnosis sometimes, but by no means always accurate. Others, like the case I have mentioned, ventured no opinion, resumé of symptoms or even location of patient or client.

It was never wise to inquire 'What is wrong with your cow?' The swift rejoinder too often was, 'That's what I want you to tell me!'

Sounds a bit trite but my colleagues tell me that it was an oft repeated dialogue and certainly a pitfall of which, even now, the newly graduated vet should be aware.

There was another problem in communication and that was establishing the location of the patient-to-be. Names like Waimamaku, Kawakawa and Punakitere — although flowing easily off the tongues of the locals — were something of a tongue-twister to a Glaswegian, even if he had had a bit of practice in coping with strange names in India while in the army. A greater problem lay with the farmers, my clients. They often seemed to feel that because they were familiar with where they lived, others should have no difficulty in finding them. Too often directions were couched in terms like, 'Up the hill — past Wilson's woolshed — house with a red roof — you can't miss it!' At that time half the houses in New Zealand had red roofs. I had noticed this from the Auckland harbour even before I had set foot on land. The other half had roofs of green.

I often missed the farmhouse in question. One point however was in my favour. The transport company where most of my messages were received was also responsible for the daily collection of cream from all over the district. Managers and drivers were fairly familiar with who lived where. Another circumstance in my favour was that I began my operations in high summer, a time as yet distant from the hectic calving season and the mud of winter. At those times delays spent in finding one's target of the moment were less than welcome.

It was very much a time for settling in. Compared with the situation later, I was not all that busy. I even had some early successes like Chappie Baldwin's heifer with the broken leg. Another case which comes to mind was that involving a very large but very lame Aberdeen Angus bull named Lochnivar, or Lochy to his friends. This bull was owned by Charlie Renwick, a fellow countryman who had emigrated from the borders of Scotland many years before. Charlie owned a fully developed, immaculately fenced property a bit to the west of Kaikohe. The bull, who wasn't all that friendly, had developed a severe infection of his right hind foot and was in considerable pain. He was thus quite unable to perform his primary function of getting the 50-odd cows in his harem in calf, a function which involved, as the reader might suspect, the temporary redistribution of the weight normally borne on four feet to only two.

Clearly Charlie was not all that optimistic.

'Been crook for a while now,' he advised, 'and you can't get near enough to him to do much with that foot. I reckon I might just have to get rid of him.'

'Considering the time lag,' I replied, 'you might have to do just that, but before you do, we might just try a new injection which works through the bloodstream without touching the foot at all.'

'I'll give anything a go,' said my client. 'This bull has left some bonny calves and I'd like to keep him if I can.'

The injection to which I referred was a sulpha drug which not too long before had almost certainly saved the life of Winston Churchill when he was stricken with pneumonia while in North Africa, and thus may have played a part in influencing the course of history. For veterinary use the drug was dispensed in two-ounce brown but transparent glass jars bearing the characteristic orange label its manufacturer used for its veterinary products. The medicine had first to be dissolved in a pint of sterile water and then — and this was the snag — injected into a vein. If injected elsewhere, without the benefit of rapid diffusion by the fast-flowing bloodstream, it could cause a very severe and even dangerous local reaction. I decided that the easiest and safest approach would be to get the patient flat on his side. He could then be restrained and it would make the large jugular vein more accessible.

I retrieved a long rope from the boot of the car. The newness of this piece of equipment did not miss Charlie's attention.

'Got some new gear as well then!' he quipped.

A fixed noose around the thick neck and a couple of half-hitches around the ribs and the flank didn't leave too much rope to spare. There was just enough room for Charlie, myself and a neighbour who had been passing, to obtain a good enough purchase. A few hefty pulls and the bull sank to his knees, rolling on to his side. Charlie, at my urgent beckoning, sat on his neck and pulled on his nose until the skin was tense near where the jugular vein rested. I clipped the hair, disinfected the skin above the vein, and with a bold thrust sought to make contact with it. A grunt of displeasure from Lochy and a scraping of boots on the ground as Charlie strove to keep his bull where we wanted him to stay, was followed by a dark fountain of venous blood from the needle. As Charlie remarked, 'I must have struck something.' I pushed the needle further into the vein. It did not take long to gravity feed the solution of the sulpha drug, remove the entangling ropes and allow a still protesting Lochy to regain his feet.

I saw the patient a week later and he was certainly a lot easier with most of the heat and pain gone from the foot. He was also once again usefully employed. However, there was understandably some deformity of the hoof. This meant that it would have to be periodically trimmed, something which was difficult but not impossible.

However all was not a bed of roses. Veterinary practice has, like most worthwhile fields of endeavour, its moments of success and even elation, interspersed with those of defeat and despair. It is to one such case I now refer; one which paradoxically involved the same sulpha drug which I had so successfully used on Charlie Renwick's bull.

I had been called to the farm of the local MP who spent most of his time concerned with affairs of state in Wellington and other places. Consequently, he arranged to have his herd milked by a sharemilker, who for a percentage of the takings, ran the farm. This was a new idea as far as I was concerned but one with which I was to become increasingly familiar. I could however, even in these early times, see the merit. The sharemilker's reward was commensurate with his effort — not a bad principle.

I was called to the farm by the sharemilker to investigate lameness in a number of the cows. On my arrival six Jersey cows were already yarded in the cowshed and all were quite severely lame. Some were even unwilling to place any weight at all on the affected foot. The feet involved were hot and painful, and clearly an acute infection was at work. It had most likely gained access through some minor damage to the skin between the claws, caused perhaps by small stones or mud which had baked hard in the sun. The condition, know as 'footrot', was a common one in the district and in spring and early summer it used to take up a good deal of my time. Later, when antibiotics became freely available, stock owners were able to successfully treat cases themselves. However, this day had not yet arrived and the best available treatment was the intravenous administration of the same sulpha drug injection I had used to treat Lochy the bull not too long before.

I explained that the drug could be a bit toxic but I little imagined that the toxicity would be at such a high level. I found that dairy cows, unlike thick-necked bulls, were good subjects for intravenous injection. Firstly they were placed in the milking bail before being securely leg-roped. Securing the hind leg prevented the milker from unwelcome kicks as they went about their business. The commodious milk vein, wending its way forward in tortuous fashion from the front of the udder, was a convenient point to enter the bovine circulation.

I administered the drug without incident and I left reasonably confident of a satisfactory outcome. My confidence was not to last! About a week later I spoke with the sharemilker from the same farm, just after finishing a very ample breakfast. He told me about a case of mastitis which sounded very much beyond repair, and this indeed proved to be the case. However, I said

I would call as apparently the sharemilker had been instructed by his absent boss to make full use of the newly installed vet. After examining the patient of the day, and giving a fairly negative prognosis, I prescribed some palliative treatment and on leaving inquired about the progress of the lame cows I had treated the week before.

'Oh them!' said the sharemilker. 'Three are good but the other three snuffed it. Like you said, that stuff you gave them can make them pretty crook!'

This was something of a shock, I can tell you, not in any way diminished by being told that the three casualties had spent the last five days underground; a post-mortem after that length of time would not have been rewarding. I wondered what had happened. The drug was acknowledged as a toxic one but it shouldn't have been that toxic. Perhaps some environmental factor could be involved? Maybe the diet had some bearing? I had had some trouble getting enough distilled water from my drug supplier to meet my needs and had been using domestic water, but only after thorough boiling and filtering. The domestic water, though, had been stored in galvanised iron tanks so perhaps there was a chemical input.

Nonetheless, the same water had been used to prepare drugs for use in other places so, while acknowledging that my technique was marginal, why had not similar problems arisen elsewhere? It was a mystery but one which did little to improve the confidence of a young practitioner. To this day the mystery remains largely unresolved. Communication on my part was clearly a problem, although I still wonder how a stock minder could accept three deaths with equanimity, not even bothering to file a report. The MP wasn't all that happy about the whole thing and felt that a bit of compensation would be in order. I believe the matter was discussed at the next meeting of the board of the dairy company but no action was forthcoming.

I subsequently arranged to collect rainwater for my injections until supplies of *aqua destillata* were regularly available.

The Administration

Apart from my veterinary work there was some administration to attend to. The veterinary committee met once a month in the RSA. hall in Ohaeawai, a wooden building with an iron roof which had started life as a domestic dwelling. After a morning session, lunch was taken in the dining room of the hotel just across the road. This was presided over with conscientious precision by a lady called Nora whose second name I never did discover. Nora was the rural equivalent of the lady in the tight black dress who controlled the affairs of the dining room in the Star Hotel in Auckland and to whom I have already made reference.

The lunch had to be arranged some days ahead and the agenda of the meetings so framed as to permit adjournment at precisely twenty-five minutes past noon. After lunch there was more debate until milking time approached, when much shuffling of feet, looking at watches and general restlessness gave notice to the chairman that it was time to call it a day. The milking of his cows dominates most days of the dairy farmer's life and no mere meeting could be allowed to interfere. I often wondered though, that if as much energy and attention as was devoted to bringing the meeting to its conclusion could have been appplied to the agenda earlier in the day, more progress could perhaps have been achieved.

The Ohaeawai Hotel was built in 1895 when the licence had been transferred from the 'public house' owned by a Mrs Wyatt-Watling at Ngawha. The licence was transferred from the site of the original 'Ohaeawai' to 'The Corner', thereafter becoming known as Ohaeawai. The hotel, which still stands, was of wide weatherboards of kauri and painted white. On the upper storey French doors opened on to a fretwork around the veranda. The top floor had a few rooms available for guests, as indeed was a requirement of the law, but the main function of the hotel was undoubtedly to quench the considerable thirst of the local and travelling public.

Ohaeawai was, and still is, a very central point situated at a junction where State Highway 1 turns abruptly right and proceeds northwards, hence the earlier name 'The Corner'. In those days the Ohaeawai sale was an important and regular feature in the farming calendar. The patrons of sales used to meet after the day's work was done to discuss their good or bad fortune. Local rugby and cricket teams with their supporters and most likely their opponents, also congregated to toast their success or drown their sorrows. I was not a great hotel drinker myself mainly because I found it difficult to get away from business in such places. It was surprising how many stock owners, stimulated by their alcoholic exuberance, suddenly seemed to recall some ailing stock way back on the farm. My 'happy hour' too often turned into an hour of consultation punctuated by a few return trips to the car for urgently needed supplies of medicines.

However, when I later became involved in local cricket I must say that I spent more than a few convivial hours in the local hostelry and even if I was often killing two birds with one stone, recollections are for the most part pleasant.

One other story concerning this hotel comes to mind, although not strictly in chronological order. When some ten years later I went farming, among the stock I took over with the farm was a very large Tamworth boar who had been around for a while. Now pigs, and boars especially, are notoriously difficult to keep in places you want them to be. The powerful snout and torpedo-like body, armoured with hide the average rhinoceros would envy, proved more than a match for all but the toughest gates and fences. My farm at that point had not reached that degree of sophistication and it was the habit of the old boar and his harem of sows to go walkabout as often as the inclination took them. Now this was not too much of a problem as long as the pigs stayed within the confines of their owner's farm, for the fences were none too flash and the pigs could easily lift the bottom wires and go about their business without causing much more damage than already existed.

In the early hours of the morning not long before Christmas, my boar decided he would carry out a bit of exploration which in the first place took him through a few of the town gardens. Perhaps he felt he too needed a holiday break. A bit of minor damage resulted but not all that serious. However, appreciating his new environment, he continued his exploration across the road and into the backyard of the hotel. In those times, beer was not on tap but delivered in glass bottles or flagons, and as might be imagined, the time before Christmas was the high point of the year for celebrations. The throughput was substantial and the empties, stacked in their crates for later return to thebrewery, grew by the hour. They formed a stack maybe twice the height of a man and half the length of a tennis court.

The boar, feeling or perhaps smelling that something interesting lay behind the mountain of empties, proceeded to investigate. He began to push with some vigour between the stack and the wall of the hotel on which it rested. Now when a boar pushes he generates a fair degree of pressure. The stack of empties had not been built to withstand that sort of leverage. The resounding crash woke management, guests and even a few semi-comatose patrons who had succumbed to the conviviality of the night before and gone to sleep in a nearby shed. The boar, sensing his unpopularity, decided to return home, but alas had been identified by someone. The next morning a none too happy licensee rang and suggested that I might like to make a small contribution towards cleaning up the havoc of the morning's early hours. I restored good public relations with an appropriate donation.

The board of the Bay of Islands Veterinary Service, my controlling authority, was originally made up of five dairy farmers. Three were from the directorate of the Bay of Islands Dairy Company and two from the smaller Kaikohe Dairy Company. They later added a sheep farmer representative — Bill Low, a Scotsman from Greenock. Sheep farmers could join the club by paying an annual subscription, and could then be accepted on the same basis as their more numerous dairy farmer colleagues.

At national level the so-called club system was co-ordinated and subsidised by a farmer-controlled organisation called the Veterinary Services Council. This in turn was government-supported and meant to control such aspects as conditions of work of the vets, provision of veterinary staff, salary levels and so on.

The Council was only partly successful and conditions of work varied enormously throughout the country. This was due to various problems including geography, availability of staff, relative wealth of the area, roading, and the attitude of controlling executives, as well as the temperament of the vets employed. In the 1950's there was an acute shortage of vets to play their part in the now booming farm industries. With no veterinary school in the country, New Zealanders wishing to enter the profession had to graduate overseas, usually in either Sydney or Brisbane. Because quotas were applied by the Australian authorities, vets like myself were recruited from the UK or elsewhere.

The co-ordinator and chief executive of the Veterinary Services Council was Alan Leslie, a Scot who was a product of the hard times between the wars. He was a true socialist whose philosophies were accepted even by farmers in the welfare state New Zealand had by now become. Leslie claimed that the club system was the only way that rural New Zealand could be served. It was a point he could easily prove as he controlled the new graduate through a system of bonding, and overseas recruits by a contract which they had to sign. This was a source of endless debate and argument.

It took me 14 years in the club system before I jumped over the wall and went out on my own. In the first year I trebled my income and retained nearly all the clients I had served in the club. It was my belief that farmers were more concerned with the quality of the service they received than the system which engendered it.

Despite staying with this system for so long I was never an enthusiast for it. I felt that such a high percentage of the profession should not be under such control. I also felt that real estate such as offices and houses should not be in the hands of controlling organisations. They should have been in the hands of the vets, who were the reason for their being there in the first place.

I thought that in those early days many of my colleagues surrendered their independence too easily. Many vets were young, over-worked, under-funded, and with newly acquired family responsibility often weighing heavily upon them. Club committees were often made up of older and more experienced men; at national level very experienced men. The vets felt something was wrong but were not sure how to go about making change. Happily, change did eventually come, although slowly. Today, where clubs do exist, they are largely under the control of vets who do the the work. I recall many hours spent at local and national meetings of the Veterinary Association discussing detail and deficiencies of current contracts. Less time would have been needed to abolish the system altogether.

A dominant figure on the Bay of Islands board was one Hubert Knox Hatrick, a veteran of Gallipoli and a commander in the more recent National Military Reserve, raised to repel any Jap intent upon crossing the shoreline of New Zealand. Hubert Hatrick was at that time deputy chairman of the Kaikohe Dairy Company, the smaller in size but not in voice of the two companies which made up my board. Hatrick defended his company's and his own viewpoint with vigour on a variety of subjects at local, regional and national level. His forthrightness had to be admired, even if a contrary viewpoint was held. An enthusiast in everything he undertook, Hatrick was a strong supporter of the vet service from the outset. He was also a successful dairy farmer in his own right and his herd often achieved the magical target of 30,000 pounds of butterfat and was thus a top performer in the district.

The annual meeting of the Kaikohe Dairy Company was an event Hatrick enjoyed and which also gave him a platform to extol the advantages and achievements of the vet service, often in terms so superlative that I personally would have found embarassing. Some suggested, perhaps unkindly, that all this was a ploy to direct attention away from the problems of the day like collection of cream, loss of cream cans and inadequate payout. Hatrick also felt that the gospel of the vet needed to be spread elsewhere. As a result he and I, with as many of the board as could be persuaded to accompany us, addressed the boards of the neighbouring dairy companies such as Whangaroa and Hokianga.

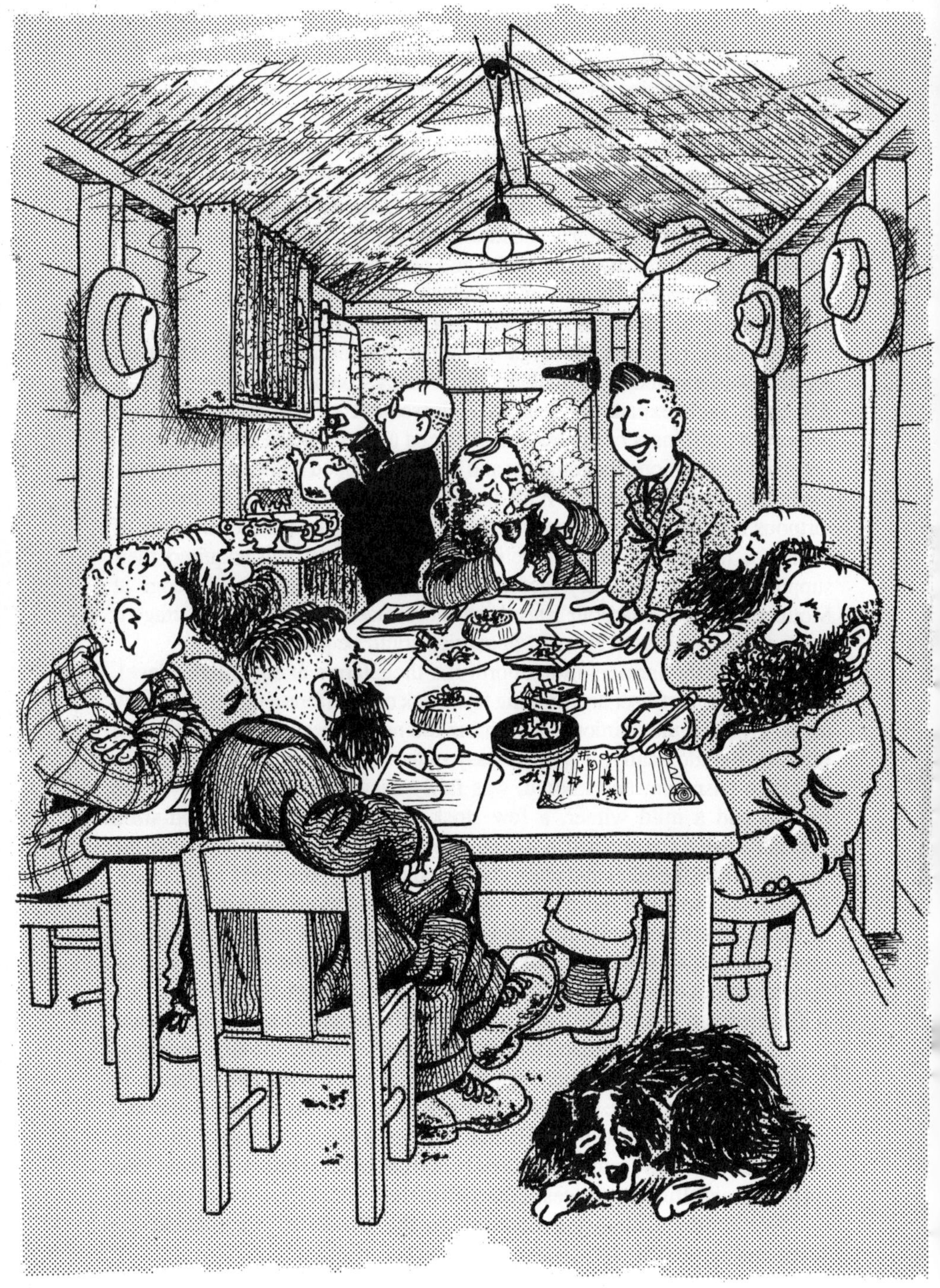

I remember paying a visit to the Oruru-Fairburns company up Mangonui way. This company had only a few suppliers with a fair proportion of them being directors. Most of these gentlemen had well-established, spade-like beards and looked to me as if they had perhaps missed out in something like 50 years of elapsed time. The board met in a discarded army hut and the officiating secretary regularly abandoned his white-collar duties to make tea, interview travellers, check the boiler and perform other sundry duties. The chairman seemed used to such interruptions and demonstrated his versatility by combining his main function with that of his secretary.

The public relations campaign was not in vain for, in time, the veterinary service was expanded to include the Whangaroa and Hokianga areas. Although such expansion was an endorsement of the acceptance and perceived usefulness of the service, it placed a heavy strain on it. The areas involved were among the roughest and least-developed in the land with poor roads and broken country. With the Hokianga bisected by its long and tortuous harbour, it presented special difficulties. Like parts of the Bay of Islands a number of farmers delivered their product and acquired their supplies by boat, the dairy factory being situated on the water's edge at Motukaraka on the harbour's northern shore. Because of a staff shortage it was a few years before any sort of service could be provided.

Many of the farmers in the north ran their farms at subsistence level, applying little fertiliser and running few stock of indifferent quality on many acres. I formed the opinion that farming did not progess as well as it might because, paradoxically, it was too easy rather than too difficult. Grass of a sort, like paspalum and kikuyu, was fairly easy to grow. With an ample rainfall and a mild winter, a few stock supplemented by a good-sized vegetable patch and orchard, not to mention eels from the creek, fish from the sea, duck from the lakes and pheasant from the brush, provided a sufficiency. Perhaps the farmer of those times was happier and more content than those of today. There was certainly always time for a cup of tea over which the topics of the day were discussed. It was often put to me that the taxation system did not encourage progress. This might have been the case but if so, it did not seem to have the same sort of psychological block further south.

Hubert Hatrick continued his crusading zeal and over the next year or so I attended a number of meetings and conferences with him relating to veterinary affairs of the club system in places as far away as Christchurch. I remember one such event in Hamilton when a farmer delegate from Te Awamutu who was seated immediately in front of us, spent quite some time on his feet extolling the virtues of that part of the country from which he came.

'We produce almost everything in the Waikato,' expounded the pompous farmer, 'butter, cheese, milk powder, beef, mutton.'

At this point, my fellow delegate, clearly fed up with the turn of events, murmured under his breath but in a still very audible whisper, 'Bull!' The orator ahead did not hear this comment clearly and interpreted it as a query, not a criticism.

'Yes,' he continued, 'and wool too.'

'I said bull!' responded a now exasperated Hatrick in a voice which reverberated around the hall, leaving none in doubt as to his meaning. The storm of laughter which ensued had a deflationary effect, causing our talkative neighbour soon to resume his seat.

Hubert Hatrick had a few eccentricities. He was good at what he did but avoided what he disliked or what he lacked competence in — not a bad formula for success when you think of it.

This was perhaps one of the reasons why he and I achieved a rapport. Farm stock suffering from any malady was clearly a mystery and one to be decentralised as soon as possible for solution. This was why I was usually summoned early and often to the Hatrick farm not far away. As a result, my success rate there was higher than in some other places and my image thus more favourable. Hatrick, perhaps because of his Irish origin, was an excellent exponent of animal husbandry and was one of the few really successful pig farmers of his time. Small male pigs had to be castrated early in life if the pork and bacon they ultimately produced was not to acquire a strong taint making it unmarketable. Most farmers performed this small operation themselves but it was not one Hatrick relished. For many years I regularly performed this task for him as batches of pigs became due. He was always convinced that this paid dividends as his mortality rate was negligible. He may have been right as it is not possible to perform surgery, however simple, while restraining a struggling subject and maintaining an acceptable standard of hygiene. As many farmers had no help, the conditions under which they operated often permitted subsequent infections, sometimes fatal. Few advertised their losses but Hatrick and I knew they happened.

There is one more tribute I must pay to Hatrick. Across the metalled road from his house he maintained a vegetable garden of nearly two acres of rich volcanic soil, a feature of the long-established settlement of Waimate North. He did this more for love than for profit, although a few rows of maize did produce a profusion of golden cobs. These were stored in a wooden shelter with slatted sides, and as occasion demanded, used to supplement the diet of his pigs. Some sugar beet and turnips served the same purpose. In later years I often returned from a visit to the Hatrick farm, the car laden with vegetables of all description; cucumber and cauliflower, cabbage and carrot, pumpkin and parsnip and many more.

I can still see on a summer's day, Hatrick with hoe in hand, hat on head, white singlet, and khaki shorts, working steadily between his prolific rows, perhaps planning some future verbal violence on an adversary at a meeting. Although we quite often disagreed, Hubert Knox Hatrick — of bald head, broad shoulders, forthright speech and steady gaze, farmer, politician (for he had once surprisingly contested the local seat for Labour), an achiever of note and integrity unquestioned — was one of my unforgettable characters.

It was time for me to take stock of the veterinary situation in the district. New Zealand is fortunate in that it has managed to steer clear of many of the animal plagues which ravage agriculture elsewhere. Foot and mouth disease, rinderpest in cattle, swine fever in pigs, scrapie in sheep, rabies in dogs to mention but a few, have mercifully kept away. This is largely because of the seas which surround this land. Man's ingenuity however, is continually contracting the time needed to move from place to place in this world of ours, so the barriers that were so effective in the past in preventing unwelcome arrivals, may not prevail forever.

Perhaps because of the absence of what may be called veterinary catastrophes, the approach to animal health problems had been somewhat muted. Few qualified advisors were available to initiate and guide programmes; and diseases which had managed to become established, flourished. The approach of farmers and others to disease problems tended to be philosophical because it was usually possible to survive while accepting a degree of loss through the ravages of stock disease. But animals and sometimes their owners did not always survive. Between 50 and 60 New Zealanders died from hydatid disease each year throughout the 1950's, and many suffered prolonged hospitalisation recovering from surgery. I suspect that an unrecorded number may have succumbed to the undulant fever caused by the brucella abortus organism which was widespread in stock at that time. The as yet unidentified leptospirosis was also probably causing severe but undiagnosed human illness.

Undulant fever and the bovine counterpart called brucellosis, or more commonly contagious abortion, was widespread where I worked. As the calving season approached it became clear to me that a significant number of cows, and more especially first-calving heifers, were not going to participate. Before the month of June was out nearly all the heifers and most of the cows in several herds had lost their calves. These cases came to my attention because following the abortion the afterbirth was commonly retained.

Farmers were philosophical, not aware that any control was possible. They were hopeful as ever, that next year things would be better. This hope was not entirely unfounded as when a herd experienced a severe abortion storm the immunity so engendered often gave a protection for a few seasons ahead. There was however a better way to impart immunity. Young calves, which received a dose of a vaccine called Strain 19 between the ages of six and eight months, developed an immunity which imparted protection for at least the first two pregnancies. This was when the problem was greatest. It was obvious that a programme of vaccination was urgently needed and my thinking and intention was that such a programme should be initiated in 1949. Even then it would be two years before any benefit could be expected as dairy heifers were usually mated as yearlings to calve a year later as two-year olds.

The presence of such widespread infection had another important implication. The disease was sometimes called Bang's disease because the bacteria causing it was first identified by a Dane of that name in 1896. The related Malta fever in man had been investigated by someone called Bruce nine years earlier and his work was acknowledged by incorporating his name into that of the bacterium he had demonstrated. Malta fever had its source in goats on the island of Malta. In humans, the illness in its simplest form, was similar to severe influenza, but with widely fluctuating body temperatures which characteristically led to it being called undulant fever. With such widespread involvement in stock it was clear to me that the disease must also have a fairly widespread human manifestation, especially as precautions such as the scalding of milk for domestic use was by no means the rule.

There were problems in diagnosis because of the similarity of the condition to flu and other common human afflictions. Positive diagnosis could only be made by demonstrating an antibody response to infection. For this to be done, a series of samples had to be sent to Dunedin, a long way away. By the time a diagnosis was confirmed the patient had usually recovered, or in odd cases, developed complications and died. Recurrence of symptoms eventuated from time to time, but they were not always related by patient or physician to the original complaint. Human infection was commonly caused through drinking infected and untreated milk, the handling of aborted foetuses, or perhaps contamination by the copious uterine discharges which usually followed abortion in the bovine. Later it was demonstrated that some freezing workers could become infected through handling infected stock. I was to become a victim myself.

Another disease which came to my attention was distemper in dogs. This was a distressing viral infection in young dogs affecting eyes, lungs and intestines and sometimes followed by fits and/or paralysis.

The death rate was high, and treatment palliative and generally unsatisfactory. Fortunately a vaccine was available and before long I was immunising dogs for miles around. In later years, regular dosing for hydatids became routine.

And so summer moved into autumn. It was less spectacular than where I came from but identifiable nonetheless—chill in the morning air, a yellowing of the poplars and a browning of the oaks. Some of these had passed into their second century, having sprung from acorns carried by sailing ships long ago.

I was well pleased with my first few months in this strange and distant land. Although most of my clients were still waiting to see me, I had already made a favourable impression on some, and had given thought to programmes of control in at least two of the animal diseases which ravaged the herds and flocks I served.

Patient and client were already better off, though neither was yet aware of it.

Home Sweet Home

The situation concerning the provision of houses in the late forties was not good. Many servicemen returning from overseas had married and needed houses. Many builders had themselves been involved in hostilities and had to regroup. The builders of the future were as yet untrained. Materials were scarce and a house of any sort was at something of a premium.

In the Veterinary Club system with which I was for the time being involved, it was customary for the employing body to supply a house where necessary for its veterinary staff. I did not particularly favour this as it encouraged an unwelcome dependency on the employer. Also any appreciation in value of the residence went to the employer and not the tenant who was the reason for the house being there in the first place.

Anyway, like it or not, that was the way things were supposed to work and so at a meeting of my board I announced my intention to marry and the consequent need for a dwelling. The announcement was greeted with the usual congratulatory ribaldry which seems to be an essential part of such disclosures. Finally the committee got down to the serious consideration of my request. The process looked like being fairly long and drawn out largely because the veterinary committee had no assets and little cash to pay for houses or anything else of value. The matter therefore had to be referred to the board of the Bay of Islands Dairy Company. However the chairman had already sustained significant losses through the activity of the newly established vet. Perhaps he felt that a longer interval should elapse before his company committed itself to providing real estate for a venture still to prove itself.

The matter was discussed by the Bay Board and it was proposed that a house might be constructed on a section on the western approach to the township of Ohaeawai. The proposed section was fairly steep and covered in a thick matt of kikuyu grass. In places, some healthy-looking gorse plants had managed to flourish. The land had at one time been the site of the first Bay of Islands Dairy Company which shifted to Moerewa in 1929. Parts of the concrete foundations still defiantly rose from the surrounding vegetation, as if a memorial to this earlier institution,

One story, which perhaps illustrates the reason why the word 'co-operative' is often incorporated in the title of dairy companies and the like, involved a director of the company. One Christmas morning he was notified that the factory had run out of coal. As a result the daily intake of cream could not be made into butter and was in some danger of being lost. The director, never one to accept defeat, ripped up several chains of fencing on his farm. He strapped the puriri posts to his horse-driven konaki and soon had them delivered to the factory. With furnaces once again stoked, business continued much as usual. No doubt the director returned home to enjoy his Christmas dinner, as well he might.

But to return to the proposed house! Tenders now had to be called and this involved a further period of inertia while any who might be interested (and there weren't many) considered a commitment. Eventually a few tenders reached the board, the lowest being one of £2,500.

'Too dear by far', unanimously resolved the board. 'We will have to think again.'

This time the thoughts turned towards the junior partner, the Kaikohe Dairy Company. Its chairman was Harold Fisher Guy, a local lawyer who was well known nationally in municipal affairs and who had a finger on the pulse of most of what was going on in the district.

Among his clients Mr Guy had an elderly nurse who lived in a house set by the road a little north of the township of Ohaeawai. The nurse felt a desire to move into town where a small flat more commensurate with her age and requirements was available for purchase. Mr Guy could see the possibility of killing two birds with the one stone. A figure of £750 was mentioned as a purchase price.

'This is more like it,' said the board. 'Our problems have been solved.'

I was naturally delighted that negotiations had taken such a positive turn, but this was before I had inspected my proposed residence. The problems of the board may have been solved but mine were only just beginning. The house, which I later discovered had been a maternity home in which a number of my clients had first seen the light of day, was situated on about two acres of mainly stony volcanic land. Through the middle of this meandered a stream. At least I presumed it meandered because it could not be seen behind a heavy screen of willow, bamboo and a canna-like weed with the simplistic name of ginger.

There was no access for vehicular traffic but a small, one-time white kauri gate opened off the road verge on a heavily metalled, dusty bend where State Highway 1 wound its way uphill towards Okaihau and places further north. The gate opened on to an overgrown path of flat rocks which skirted the jungle hiding the creek, and which led to the dwelling.

I moved cautiously round the veranda, which enclosed the house on two sides, and approached what I took to be the back door. I rapped lightly to announce my presence. This was met with a sort of scraping, scuffling and splashing from within as if someone was in a hurry; perhaps getting out of the bath? After a further interval the door was partially opened by a little old lady who asked my business. In the background on the sink bench, or it would have been if there had been a sink, I noticed a number of used cans sporting labels like baked beans and pineapple. I deduced later that these cans were strategically placed around the kitchen floor when rain fell as the iron roof had a number of defects. When visitors threatened, the cans were quickly collected and stored until further rain fell. It was the hurried collection of these cans which explained the strange sequence of noises I had heard.

It must be remembered that at this point I was no prospective buyer — only a possible tenant and this status did not place me high in the estimation of my erstwhile hostess. However, after a bit of discussion I was admitted and had my first look at my residence-to-be.

The kitchen was a lean-to, supported by the older part of the house which consisted of two fairly orthodox sections. They looked as if they might have been built separately and then joined together. Each section had it own basic roofing system and the roofs met at the bottom of a 'V' which I later discovered was, in the trade, called a valley. This valley was supposed to catch the rain-water from roughly half the house but it was too shallow and had inadequate fall. The result was that when the rain fell and the wind blew, some water usually found its way into a bedroom below, indicated by peeling wallpaper and a growth of healthy-looking mould underneath. Apart from the kitchen roof and these two defects apart, the place seemed reasonably waterproof.

The weatherboards, which also looked as if they could have been improved by a few coats of paint, were of wide kauri. They had withstood the ravages of time and weather for perhaps 70 years, paint or no, and seemed likely to survive for some time yet. Some of the puriri blocks holding the place up had not survived, but the original builder had obviously taken their lifespan into consideration. Where volcanic boulders were handy he had used them as a pile. As a result the floors sloped a bit here and there but nothing too serious. With four bedrooms and two lounges there was no lack of space. However the problems were with the water supply and sanitation. The main water supply drained off half the house, or what I euphemistically called the east wing. It then drained onto the kitchen roof which then added its quota, less what fell directly into the kitchen below.

Finally the water drained into two square 400-gallon tanks, which I later found out had been primarily used in earlier times to protect the considerable loads of china during the long voyage from Britain to New Zealand. The contents of these sturdy tanks constituted most of the domestic supply. One tap supplied the kitchen, and because there was no sink the water was collected in an enamel basin for dishwashing and the like. The other tap supplied water to the bathroom, a sort of annex to the kitchen whose chief furnishings seemed to be another basin and a bath of galvanised iron.

The laundry was in a tin shed outside and its water supply was from a fairly rusty iron tank precariously perched on a platform supported by four puriri posts. Their diameter was being steadily reduced at and below ground level by the ravages of time. Kauri wooden wash tubs stood in one corner and in another sat a copper. This was enclosed in concrete with a firebox below.

The toilet was a long-drop model — virtually a septic tank without any refinements like outlets or inlets. But the hole had been dug deep and true and the volcanic soil provided excellent drainage. All it needed was a bit of spraying now and then to keep the flies away and freshen the atmosphere.

The house had one feature which interested me. Off the veranda opened a narrow door leading into a narrow room. Could this be my future surgery?

If you concluded that the residence left a lot to be desired then you would be right but do not altogether blame the owners. Remember the north was a bit of a backwater and had just been through years of slump and war — not exactly the climate for exotic real estate to spring up all over the place. After all, the house even had electric power and at 26-years old one is a visionary. As I walked down the path of stones towards the road and my car, my imagination was at work already planning what could be. Some noble oaks clad in autumn glory towered above the willow and bamboo, and there was a sense of tranquility broken only by the bell-like sound of a tui in a nearby tree. It was as though he was bidding me a welcome or maybe a warning!

At this point it became clear that considerable effort and expense was going to be needed to make the place acceptable to me, not to mention a new wife, but when I put the matter before the board the response was muted. There would be none of the heavy input of capital that the house needed.

I have never been a particularly patient sort of individual and I felt frustration starting to well within me again. Following the maxim of 'boldness be my guide' — one which all Scots do not regularly practise — I surprised the board by offering to buy the place myself if that would preserve the finances of the local dairy industry and assuage its conscience. Surprisingly, my suggestion was not accepted with the alacrity I had expected. However, after a few more meetings and discussions it was agreed that the option would be transferred to me. I was at last to become one of the landed gentry.

During my army service I had managed to accumulate some £800, most of which I had obtained while in India where allowances were high and expenses light. What I had in the Bank of New South Wales in Kaikohe would be enough to buy the place and even start on some sort of renovation programme. I now started negotiations with the elderly owner who, of course, had to have her new abode in Kaikohe set up before vacating the one in which she now lived. A problem which weighed heavily upon her was the fact that she had too much furniture which could not be fitted into her smaller residence-to-be. To solve this problem and to encourage her departure, I purchased a variety of items from her for £24. Not only did I now own a house and two acres but a rimu chest of drawers, a small table of the same timber, a couple of beds with only one mattress, a settee and squab (new word for me), a kitchen table, a Chinese table with bamboo legs and a miscellaneous collection of cutlery, crockery, pots and pans.

I naturally wanted to get things moving and I felt that the Baldwins with whom I boarded, would also welcome my departure. They were not landlords at heart and the invasion of their privacy was something I wanted to end. I was also monopolising their telephone as my business grew and they could hardly, so to speak, get a word in edgeways.

It was all very well to shift, but how about things like food and laundry? I wasn't much of a cook by inclination and with the calving season fast approaching I could see my time for domestic duties might be limited. As is usually the case, if you look hard enough something will turn up. For me the solution lay with a family who operated the local village forge and engineering workshop.

Alec Anderson had come to New Zealand from his native Glasgow some years before and he told me in an accent as broad as the day he had sailed down the Clyde, that before he left that city he had worked with one Donald Campbell. Campbell was a well-known veterinary surgeon at a time when most of the veterinary work related to the horse, which in peace and war was the main means of transportation. Many of the problems with horses between the wars involved their feet and it was important that vet and blacksmith established a rapport. Often shoes had to be removed to identify injury or disease in the foot, and sometimes special shoes had to be made to protect sensitive structures or avoid injury to a leg. Alec and his two sons operated their business with skill and success often interspersed by vigorous debate between themselves and their clients, who found the blacksmith's shop an agreeable spot to spend a bit of time while their horse was being shod or machinery repaired. Not only were horses shod but the firm claimed with some truthfulness that they would repair anything but the break of day.

It was decided that I would have my evening meal with the Andersons, and the lady of the house kindly consented to do my laundry. This was a task which, as the calving season progressed, she must have found fairly daunting even if used to dealing with the dirty clothes of her all-male engineering family. However, in my case the dirt was often of animal origin and of a type she may not have known before.

Towards the beginning of winter I said my farewells and thanks to the Baldwins and took over the key of my new dwelling, metaphorically speaking. Actually the key had been lost, most likely years before. This was not important as burglaries were unheard of and most houses were left unlocked when their owners were away. In any case, I didn't have a lot to interest the average thief.

At my solicitor Ken Harold's office in Kaikohe I signed the necessary documents and handed over my cheque. Home at last!

I was now faced with the task of renovation. An oft quoted saying is that the thing to do is to get an old place and do it up. I have now been involved in this technique at least three times and am still not sure of its wisdom. This was my first attempt and probably the most dramatic, undertaken at a time when labour and materials were at a premium and often of indifferent quality. It was not so much a question of engaging tradesmen as persuading them to perform. I was lucky. There lived at nearby Pakaraka a worthy called Eric Walker, an ex-farmer who on retirement took on jobs around the place, mainly as a plumber. I don't think he had any trade certificate but in those days that was of little consequence.

The main thrust of the plumbing operation was to establish a high tank on a stand above roof level and install an electric pump which would deliver water from the nearby creek into the tank. Fortunately the creek briefly appeared from its enclosing jungle near the corner of the house and a downpipe from the pump could easily be submerged at that point. For drinking water it was decided to retain the two square tanks which Eric had pronounced sound, but only after he had sealed a leak in one with a half-pound of black bitumastic compound called Hydroseal. It was a system which served us well for 13 years, and apart from the odd blocked foot valve was largely trouble-free.

The roof above the leaking kitchen needed to be renewed but items like roofing iron, toilet pans, hand basins and so on had much in common with hens' teeth. I had to use my influence with as many board members as would listen to obtain them through the trading department of the Bay Dairy Company. Like other retailers they received only a quota of such items at that time.

For a carpenter I found an elderly tradesman called Jack Ireland, who lived in Kaikohe. Jack set to work with a will, first of all building a tank stand on a solid concrete foundation already laid by Eric Walker. He next turned his attention to the lining of the kitchen, which being liberally peppered with borer holes needed to be concealed with hardboard. A kauri benchtop was obtained from somewhere and in it set an enamel sink with a greenish hue. Soon the taps were installed — one hot, one cold for the creek water, and one in the middle for drinking water from the rain-water tanks.

A septic tank was of course a necessity and this was installed by a drain layer from Kaikohe who had a tough sort of a job digging a big hole through the rocky ground. The same man showed his versatility by building a new brick fireplace in lounge number one and another in lounge number two. Examination had revealed a charring of the timber surrounding the existing fireplaces, indicating how close the old place must have come to going up in smoke in its latter years. As new owner, I was anxious to avoid this. Eric and Jack added another lean-to housing a toilet and shower, something of an innovation in that part of the world at that time. Further consultation with my bride-to-be indicated a desire to improve the laundry facilities. I had met an ex-serviceman cum carpenter/builder called Fred Paul at the Kawakawa races, an annual event then held in summer on a dried-out swamp on the outskirts of the town. I managed to persuade him to construct the new washhouse as a further annex to the kitchen.

One more jewel had yet to be added to my collection of tradespeople which I had painstakingly assembled. As might be imagined, extensive interior decorating was needed. The exterior needed even more attention but I had resolved to carry that out myself at some later time. The wallpaper in three of the four bedrooms was in reasonable order although of a pattern I myself would not have chosen. The paper in bedroom four was a disaster badly affected by water from the valley above.

The paper in the lounges had a background of dark green on which embossed rose-pink impressions of triffid-like plants embraced each other in an ill-conceived pattern. This was all a bit much and I decided that replacement with a paper of more conservative design would be in order. This was a job for the expert as it was not just a matter of sticking the paper on the wall. The lining of the rooms was of irregular rough-sawn kauri board, and on these strips of hessian needed to be tacked through bands of narrow tape to provide a surface for receiving the wallpaper. The laying and tightening of this scrim, as it was called, was a task calling for expertise. If not properly done the occasional draught which always used to penetrate these old houses caused the scrim and wallpaper to billow back and forth alarmingly, rather like the sail of some ship at sea.

I found the man for the job in 83-years old Teddy Jones, a tradesman who had never retired. He was well versed in the ways of scrim, paper and paint.

When he came to paint the ceiling of the lounge using a four inch brush, he used no protective covering on the floor so I was apprehensive lest the not unattractive kauri boards would be forever spotted. I need have had no fear as ne'er a drop was spilled.

It must not be assumed that the momentous events to which I have referred took place in a matter of days or even weeks or that they proceeded in the order in which I have presented them. Things proceeded as people and materials were available. Sometimes for days on end peace prevailed while timber and tools and plumbers' pipes lay undisturbed. Suddenly the place would spring to life and the smell of new-sawn timber and the tang of fresh paint encouraged my optimism.

Even when I left for the celebration of my wedding some six months later Teddy Jones was still applying 'knotting' to the cupboard doors and Eric Walker yet another half-pound of Hydroseal to another leak he had discovered in one of the water tanks.

The Busy Season

In America and most of Europe nearly all the milk produced goes directly to consumers in the towns and cities, making it necessary to maintain a constant supply all year round. In New Zealand only a small proportion of the national dairy herd is so orientated. The rest of dairying is concerned with converting milk into products like butter, cheese and milk powder. As such products can be stored and sold later, the industry concentrates its productive effort through spring and early summer when the growth of grass is usually most prolific. This factor has made this country one of the leaders in grassland farming and the marketing of products emanating from this form of agricultural endeavour.

The impact of all this on the country veterinary surgeon is significant for it means that there is a concentration of calving cows, lambing ewes and associated problems during the months of July, August and September. While calving is said to take place in the spring it actually happens in the middle of winter when the weather is at its most inclement.

Although I had been warned of storms ahead I had yet to have that experience. Meanwhile, life proceeded in a relatively leisurely fashion.

One bit of progress I had fortunately made was the acquisition of a surgery. I have already referred to the possibilities in this direction of the small room which opened through a narrow door off the veranda of my new home. These possibilities now began to be translated into reality. Jack Ireland managed to produce another kauri bench and constructed a battery of cupboards on one wall and drawers and shelves on another. More cupboards below the sink and a Zip heater for hot water followed. A small rimu table I had purchased as part of my package deal with the former lady owner of the house, served as an operating table for small animals. Eventually I had this table covered in stainless steel; it was rather too small for the job but the size of the room did not permit anything bigger and it served its purpose for 13 years.

I was acquiring luxuries in a professional sense which had not previously been my lot, and when Teddy Jones applied the finishing touch with a few coats of white enamel it all looked quite smart. Although the place by today's standards would be considered quite inadequate, many were the operations I performed in that small room. Many gallons of calcium injection, pounds of stomach powder, and thousands of scour pills for ailing calves were dispensed within its walls. The surgery was also a forum for discussion and debate with farmers, veterinary students, drug salesmen and others who stopped by, mostly on business but sometimes for pleasure.

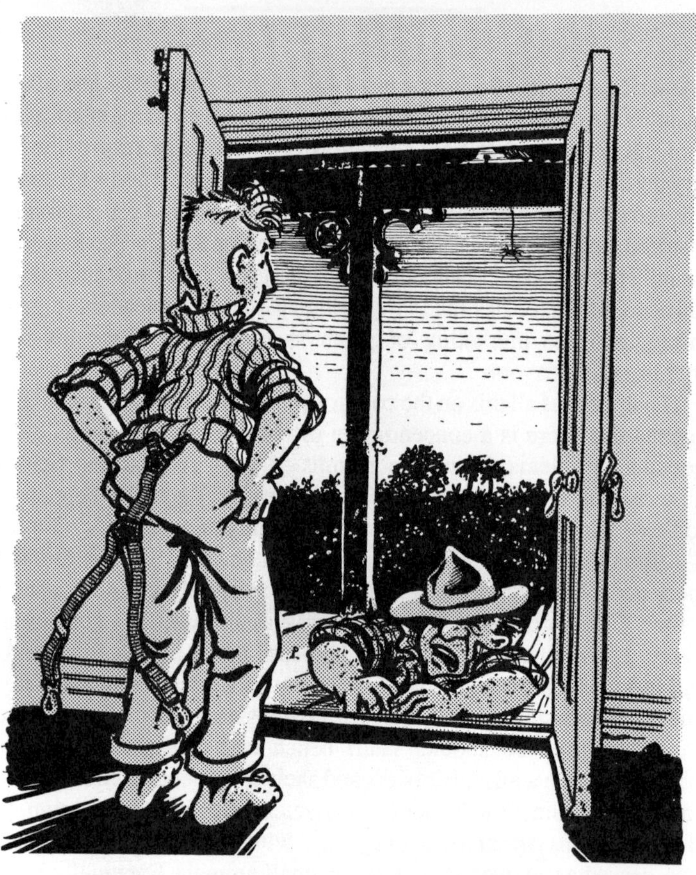

There was one incident concerning the surgery which, I suppose, was a bit of a catastrophe at the time, but in retrospect has its funny side. It hadn't taken the farmers too long to find out where the medicines they needed for their stock were kept and from the beginning they often called in person to collect supplies. One morning while still in bed I heard the clump of heavy feet on the veranda onto which the French doors of my bedroom opened. I hastily pulled on some trousers. I was about to open the door when the clump of footsteps abruptly ended, only to be succeeded by a loud crash of breaking timber, a further thump, then silence, but only for a moment. A number of expletives followed, comforting only to the extent that it confirmed that no fatality had taken place.

I opened the French door and noticed a wartime soldier's hat atop a head, along with a pair of muscular shoulders protruding from a large hole in the veranda floor. Assisting my client from his temporary hideaway I explained that the veranda had a fair degree of borer infestation and that it was my medium-term intention to do something about it. I expressed the hope that he was uninjured.

As we cautiously proceeded towards the door of the surgery he replied, 'No sweat there mate, but maybe for now you should put up a notice *Beware of the borer* — or something like that!'

I said I would give his advice consideration.

One feature of the district was the considerable variation in soil types and topography. This had a significant influence on the calving pattern as far as its timing was concerned. Ohaeawai was surrounded by a number of imposing volcanoes, happily long extinct. The mainly volcanic soil was mostly reddish but occasionally black, liberally interspersed by boulders of varying dimension. These had been projected in violent storms from the surrounding peaks. It was one such boulder, named *Taiamai*, which I have described in the preface. Situated near the Ohaeawai township, it was named by the Maoris of long ago. In time this respected stone gave its name to the whole district.

These volcanic soils were rich in some minerals, and they were porous and free-draining, allowing the copious rainfall of winter and spring to pass through to reservoirs and rivers far below. The soils responded quickly to the change of seasons. The growth of ryegrass was well-established before June came to its end. Farmers on the volcanic belt took advantage of this and had their cows calve early in June. There was further wisdom in this policy because if the weather became dry and hot as it often did, a good proportion of the season's production had already been secured. Once the weather became dry and hot the grass failed to grow and the grazing cows responded with an often dramatic fall-off in production. The belt of volcanic land was limited, reaching only as far as Pakaraka in the south and Kaikohe to the west, with smaller areas around Waimate North and at Kerikeri out towards the east coast.

The rest of the area I covered was variable, but essentially of heavy clay. There were some river flats, such as in the Waihou Valley. A river of the same name flowed through the valley, soon to expand into the long and tortuous Hokianga Harbour which meets the sea near Opononi. This valley was also of interest to me as it contained the earthworks, and indeed some station platforms, of a railway system which was intended to link the northern terminus at Okaihau with points further north. The project was set up as a means to provide employment during the Depression years, but it was abandoned before completion. The relics, still preserved, stand as some sort of memorial to the line that never was.

In such heavy land the rains of winter took longer to disperse, and the premature calving of cows and consequent traffic from milking shed to pasture would have resulted in the creation of a veritable quagmire.

I often admired the panorama provided by this Waihou Valley as I had a number of clients who farmed on a plateau on its western rim. To the east on fine days the sun reflected on the silver river, while early mornings saw the bush-clad hills visible above an all-enshrouding morning mist. They were like islands in some strange and silent sea.

Paradoxically, for all its beauty, it was this river which placed my life in danger for possibly the first, but certainly by no means the last time, during my years in veterinary practice.

I had received a written message via the cream can — not an unusual way to transmit and receive messages or take delivery of small stores in those days. The thrust of the message was that a Maori farmer who lived across the river, owned stock which was dying at regular intervals and in significant numbers. He needed urgent advice. Would I phone an Okaihau number. I thought all this un-necessarily ponderous but when I rang that evening I could see the reason for the need to plan. Although the line was far from perfect I learned that the river was in partial flood from recent rain. Even if I attended when the tide in the Hokianga was on ebb there would be problems getting across.

The river could be forded fairly easily in odd places where banks of shingle sloped gently towards the stream, but this did not apply under conditions of flood. In other places, bridges of timber cross-pieces supported by number 8 fencing wire, had been anchored to willows or other convenient trees. Sadly none of these served the needs of my client-to-be, who indicated to me that if I could attend around ten the next morning the tide would be on ebb. He would meet me with a horse, skilled at negotiating the river even when in flood.

All this sounded fairly adventurous, and it looked a bit more than that when I arrived the next day to find a foam-flecked torrent about 30 yards wide rushing madly towards the sea. My client, a Maori of middle age and gentle eye, was clad in a sou'wester and a long, oiled, water-proof drover's coat. With his boots on the far bank to ensure that they stayed dry, he had arrived with not one but two horses, explaining that a load of two people would be a bit much for one under the prevailing conditions.

My client explained the technique for gaining the far bank. There were three departure and arrival points — two on the side of his farm and one on the side on which we now stood. Point one on the far side was upstream and allowance had to be made for the current, for the horse had to swim a fair part of the middle section of the river. Point two was about 40 yards downstream where arrival could be reasonably expected. Similarly, in the reverse direction, the current again had to be considered and an arrival point on a shingle bank another 40 yards away downstream was the target.

'But,' added my client, 'by golly be sure you don't miss that shingle bank, cause after that the river goes into a gully and if you get in there you won't stop till you get to Opononi!'

I was no stranger to horses, having had more than my quota of riding experience in the army — everything from dressage to chasing gazelles across the dusty plains of the Punjab. But swimming horses across flooded rivers was something new. My horse, perhaps not yet used to the white man's ways, eyed me with suspicion as I climbed aboard, boots suspended round my neck where I hoped they would stay dry. If they didn't it wouldn't matter much because I wouldn't be needing them any more! My client and erstwhile guide promptly grabbed my bag and mounted his steed. No doubt keen to get home, his steed plunged into the torrent in a cloud of spray, and mine, not to be outdone, quickly followed. Soon the sensation of being supported by four legs changed to being supported by none as buoyancy was gained and swimming began.

I could see what my client had meant as the current took over and our course became distinctly more diagonal. I could see too, the approach of the steep-sided chasm through which the river churned with increasing violence just beyond our projected point of arrival. Would I make it or drown at sea or, more likely, long before I reached there? My steed, however, knew his business, and in a manner similar to Tam o' Shanter's mare, reached a safe haven. With relief I again felt hooves make contact with terra firma.

I discovered that the most likely cause of my client's worry lay in the fact that early in autumn he had set fire to a steep hillside covered in bracken fern. The rains since had caused a multitude of new, brown, healthy-looking fronds to push their way out of the blackened embers. As grass for the cows had started to diminish with colder and wetter weather, he decided to save as much as he could by grazing a mob of about 20 young heifers on the burn-off. After about three weeks the heifers had started to die and he had lost six. The one I saw, which had apparently died only that morning, showed all the signs of fern poisoning, including bleeding from the bowel and small pinpoint haemorrhages on the pale membrane lining the eyes and mouth.

I advised my client to get his stock off the fern without delay and keep them away for at least three weeks, and even then only allowing them back on a week-on, week-off basis.

'Too right!' responded the farmer. 'Can't beat the pakeha for getting to the bottom of a man's trouble. How'd you fancy a bit o' wild pork for your tea?'

I thanked him for his offer but explained that I was not yet my own cook; perhaps another time?

'I might have to get you back again if I have any more trouble, eh?'

I said that I hoped the river would be more tranquil if and when that happened.

The return journey appeared marginally less hazardous, perhaps because the threatening gully was not so near this time, or maybe I was just getting better at it!

In such heavy country, seasonal calving was often delayed until August or September. It was thus possible to attend to most of the veterinary problems involving stock on the earlier country before the heavier land had started to pour forth its seasonal bounty of new life.

The impact of calving had begun even before I left the Baldwins. One morning, Eric, already some hours into his day, banged on my bedroom door and said he had a cow down. I threw on some clothes and picked up some gear from the boot of the car before accompanying him towards his cowshed. We crunched across paddocks already white with an early frost, while the light of day enhanced by the tip of the sun appearing over the eastern hills, grew steadily stronger. The cow was, in technical jargon, in lateral recumbency, but in more descriptive terms — flat out. I gathered that Jersey, Annie, had calved the day before and it wasn't too difficult to arrive at a diagnosis of milk fever.

Milk fever was a condition which was to occupy a good deal of my time in the busy season every year. The chemistry is most likely quite complicated but is most easily understood by appreciating that in the blood of the normal cow and other species there is a very small but very necessary amount of calcium present. When a cow calves this calcium tends to be drawn off, in part to provide the considerable quantities of that element present in milk, provided in abundance to meet the needs of the newly-born calf and her farmer owner. The blood shortfall is made up by a compensatory withdrawal from the bovine bones but, alas, in some cases the compensation is too slow and too late. The result is that the calcium in the blood falls to as low as one third of what it ought to be.

The symptoms of milk fever are a result of the fall in blood calcium and chiefly involve the nervous system. Early on there is staggering with a tendency to follow the line of least resistance — downhill. The affected animal soon sits down and may appear normal. But careful inspection may reveal an s-shaped bend in the neck, the consequence perhaps of some uneven muscular spasm. In time, maybe feeling sleepy, the victim settles on her side. The victim goes into a coma and if left untreated, dies.

The chief danger to life in milk fever cases was delay in treatment and the geography of the place of onset. If treatment was delayed until coma supervened, the muscular relaxation often allowed stomach contents to pass up the gullet into the throat. Undigested grass passed into the lungs could bring about a serious and usually fatal pneumonia. This progressed to its termination even if the original milk fever was completely cured. As I have said, staggery milk fever cases usually followed the line of least resistance and that was downhill. Fences seemed no barrier and as water often flowed or collected at the bottom of hills, death through drowning or chilling was by no means uncommon.

There was still a great deal of confusion among my clients concerning milk fever. It must be remembered that because of slump and war the application of lime and superphosphate had, in the north at least, been minimal. As a result the fast-growing, protein-rich ryegrass and clover was not yet the rule, although things were changing rapidly. It was such pastures which stimulated early milk flow and thus encouraged the onset of milk fever and other problems. Many farmers, often encountering milk fever for the first time, regarded it as some form of incurable paralysis. Others, through their reading or the tales of their friends, were aware of the condition but resorted to the earlier treatment of inflation of the udder. This rather curious treatment, slightly reminiscent of witchcraft, was carried out by blowing up all four quarters of the udder via the teats using a bicycle pump. The teats were then tied off with a ligature to prevent the escape of air. Strange it may seem this treatment was advised in early veterinary literature. In some cases it seemed to produce a result, perhaps by causing a temporary check to milk production and consequent loss of blood calcium. However, often the air pressure was inadequate and the ligatures not applied tightly. This led to escape of the air or strangulation and subsequent gangrene of the teats.

The use of unsterilised equipment sometimes led to the introduction of infection, resulting in severe mastitis or inflamation of the udder. All in all I don't think that too many cases were cured by this method — not where I lived anyway. The introduction of calcium by injection revolutionised the treatment. In many cases it appeared almost a miracle when a cow, apparently almost on the threshold of death, was on her feet and again of this world within a few minutes of replacing the deficient element from the bottle.

There is no doubt that the reputation I established in my early days was as much as anything due to the spectacular response to the injection of calcium in uncomplicated cases of milk fever. Being the first in the district to use the intravenous injection of calcium, endowed me with an enormous psychological and professional advantage.

But to get back to Baldwin's Annie. She lay on her side but as I walked round her she followed me with her eye. The occasional switch of her tail told me that coma had not yet set in, so a favourable prognosis was in order.

'What's all the panic, Eric?' I asked. 'Its only a milk fever; she'll be on her feet in a couple of shakes once I get some calcium into her.'

Here I was taking something of a chance. Sometimes cows, Jerseys in particular, seemed determined to die. They remained stubbornly recumbent even when the treatment administered suggested that recovery should have been swift and sure. Staying down in the open, in the mud and cold of winter, was a luxury no animal could afford. The chilling effect soon penetrated the muscles of locomotion, and proved fatal.

Annie had no such psychological hang-up. True to prediction, when the prescribed dose of calcium borogluconate had flowed by gravity into her circulation and restored her depleted reserve, she was rolled into a sitting position. A gentle tap with my boot on her rear encouraged her to regain her feet. A trifle unsteady she made her way towards her mates waiting bunched together by the gate leading to Highway 1. The highway was used as a race along which stock could be driven to reach the more distant part of the farm.

'You know,' commented my client-landlord, 'last year I lost three cows like that just after they calved.'

His disbelief at the remarkable recovery of his cow was plain to see. Being a pioneer had some advantages.

Although milk fever was one condition the successful treatment of which could enhance a reputation with little effort, the same could not be said in relation to the calving cow, or rather the one that couldn't. My experience in this field was at that time limited and confined to my student days in Lanarkshire in Scotland, where students were not encouraged to practice anything that was too difficult and risky for fear that the reputation of the practice might be compromised.

I had also had a bit to do with the problems besetting the calving cow in India where I was in veterinary charge of a large holding complex made up of some 2,000 head of cattle and 10,000 sheep and goats. The idea was to assemble this large mass of livestock over a wide area on behalf of the Indian

Army. This allowed a period of quarantine to permit such diseases as foot and mouth, rinderpest, pleuro-pneumonia of goats and so on to get themselves out of the system. The animals were then sent forward in small batches of hopefully healthy stock by way of the Bengal and Assam Railway to Burma and north-east India. The British and Indian troops were still in conflict with the Japanese, and they appreciated some fresh meat in their diet. The Indians were very partial to curry and rice as a means of sustenance. Field butcheries converted the livestock to food as near as possible to where it was to be consumed. Refrigeration facilities were not available and in the generally hot and humid conditions meat could not be left lying around for long.

It so happened that a small proportion of the cattle bought by contractors was found to be pregnant and were kept until they calved. The milk from our unofficial dairy herd was a welcome supplement to the diet of the soldiers charged with the running of the cattle control unit. In such a herd there was the occasional problem relating to calving and I usually dealt with these. It was useful experience without having to worry about client reaction.

I remember on one occasion during my morning inspection coming upon a number of my subordinate Indian veterinary officers arranged in a semicircle around a cow confined in a staunchion. From the vagina there protruded two legs belonging to a calf still inside. My colleagues, one of whom was resting on a polo stick, were instructing a small inoffensive-looking *sowar*, or private soldier, in the handling of bovine dystokia. He didn't appear to be making much progress, maybe because it was his first attempt. The Indian officers clearly considered that their status precluded any personal intervention, particularly if soiling of the hands or clothing appeared likely. When I threw off my bush coat, soaped an arm and plunged it into the depths of the bovine uterus, their surprise and consternation was clear to see. I soon had a minor deviation of the head corrected and a healthy calf dropped by a grateful mother. I hoped it was a lesson to my reluctant colleagues that the boss often should be a participant as well as an administrator. It was a principle that, alas, was not too often practiced on the sub-continent of India.

But a herd of 30 cows in India in 1945 was not the same as one maybe 500 times as big in the Bay of Islands three years later. The main problem in calving was that many cows were looked after by few people. This permitted relatively cheap production and facilitated marketing. It did not generally encourage regular and close supervision. Cows at grass tended to fall into some sort of vacuum when darkness fell. Overnight, the calf and sometimes the mother had been lost through inattention. Some farmers, armed with probing searchlight, made a pre-bedtime inspection of their stock, but few wanted to return to their workplace at that hour. It was a step I advocated from the beginning, and carried out myself when I later went farming.

One superficial blessing of this was that the calls I received after dark were a lot less frequent than in Britain. There, after attending a dance or the cinema, farmers often discovered they needed veterinary attention late at night. The cowshed, or byre as it was called, often opened off the kitchen and it was easy to check the stock at any hour of the night or day. Although night calls for me were not usual, the deterioration in the patient's condition often made my task the next day much more difficult.

The nature of some of the complications should perhaps be explained. Normal birth in the bovine depends upon the head of the calf nestling between the forelegs, with its nose just above the knees pointing in the same direction towards the outside world. With the calf in this position it is a comparatively easy matter for the uterine contractions of the mother, aided by the contraction of her powerful abdominal muscles, to summarily expel her progeny with ease. If the head becomes twisted to one side, or one or both forelegs point in the wrong direction, the transverse diameter of the calf becomes greater than that of the mother's bony pelvis. Birth becomes impossible. Sometimes the calf is back to front and birth may proceed only if the hind legs are fully extended backwards.

If not, the transverse diameter through the hips becomes too great for the calf to proceed into its new world. Another problem was calves that were too big or mothers which were too small. Two-year-old Friesian heifers tend to have calves on the large side. Bulls on the loose often resulted in heifers sometimes becoming pregnant before they were due.

One important complicating factor lay in the bovine pelvis where the various nerves supplying the hind limbs had their origin in various clusters, leaving the bony spinal column just above the uterus. When the calf was not promptly delivered the powerful but vain expulsive efforts of the mother caused a crushing and bruising of these nerves between the inflexible bones of the mother above and those of her offspring below. This led to a temporary, or occasionally permanent paralysis and consequent loss of control of the hind legs. Now it is one thing to deliver a calf when the mother is standing up, but quite another when she is not. For instance, there was the problem of manipulating a badly deviated head of a large Friesian calf within a smallish heifer unable or unwilling to stand. It might occur on a wet Saturday afternoon in August when the farmer owner had gone to the football leaving a willing but not so strong wife temporarily in charge.

Many an hour I've spent lying on the concrete of cowsheds or sometimes in the mud. The ground grew harder and the clothes wetter by the minute, as a conglomeration of uterine fluids, watery lubricants and often rain, managed to find its way into the best of protective clothing. This is why I always preferred to attend my patients late at night, rather than sleep on it and have my problems compound for the next day.

Among my early clients was a brother and sister from the Emerald Isle. Even though they had lived in New Zealand for many years they still followed many of the ways of their ancestors. The kitchen of their home into which I was regularly invited for a cup of tea, was also often the home of a miscellaneous collection of animals and poultry. Care had to be taken before one sat down, lest a nesting hen or newly laid eggs had claimed prior occupancy.

Mick and Sarah lived across a stream prone to flooding. They were sometimes isolated for days at a time as the timber and fencing wire bridge disappeared downstream with the flood. Luckily, the bridge soon became entangled in the prolific willows lining the banks and was fairly easily recovered and re-erected.

Ducks waddled from creek to kitchen picking up any titbits they could find. I recall a black cat with a litter of bonny black and white kittens. Their eyes were still unopen, and they were asleep on an old horse hair settee by the fireside while I was accorded a bit of old Irish hospitality at the table.

Mick and Sarah milked a small herd of highly producing Jersey cows. Their pastures were regularly manured with lime and superphosphate resulting in a flush of ryegrass and clover in the spring. As well as encouraging the herd to produce at well above average levels it also inevitably produced the odd case of milk fever. Most of the farm was on flat land reached by a track which pursued a zigzag course up the hillside behind the cowshed and the house. The house had been built on a small area of flat on the bank of the creek. To provide enough space for the house, part of the steep hillside had in days gone by been excavated, leaving the back of the house tucked in close to an overhanging bank.

As I made my way across the swaying bridge in which I never did have complete confidence, I could see a worried-looking Mick awaiting my arrival on the other side.

'This cow had just had a calf to that good bull I bought last year,' Mick informed me. 'She was alright last night for I went up and had a look at her with me lamp just before bed' His accent wouldn't have been amiss in Galway or Connemara.

I picked up my bag and started up the track.

'Sure, but she's not up there,' said Mick

'Where then,' I enquired, 'does she happen to be?'

'Well, to be sure, she's on the kitchen roof,' replied Mick.

This astonishing piece of information caused me to pause and reconsider.

'How,' I asked ' did she get up there?'

I was told that Mick's cow, as milk fever cases do, had staggered

downhill from the plateau above, through a couple of sparsely wired fences
— for fencing was not one of Mick's stronger points — and as the roof of the
lean-to kitchen was within a very few feet of the sloping bank behind, had
ended up, as Mick had said, on the kitchen roof.

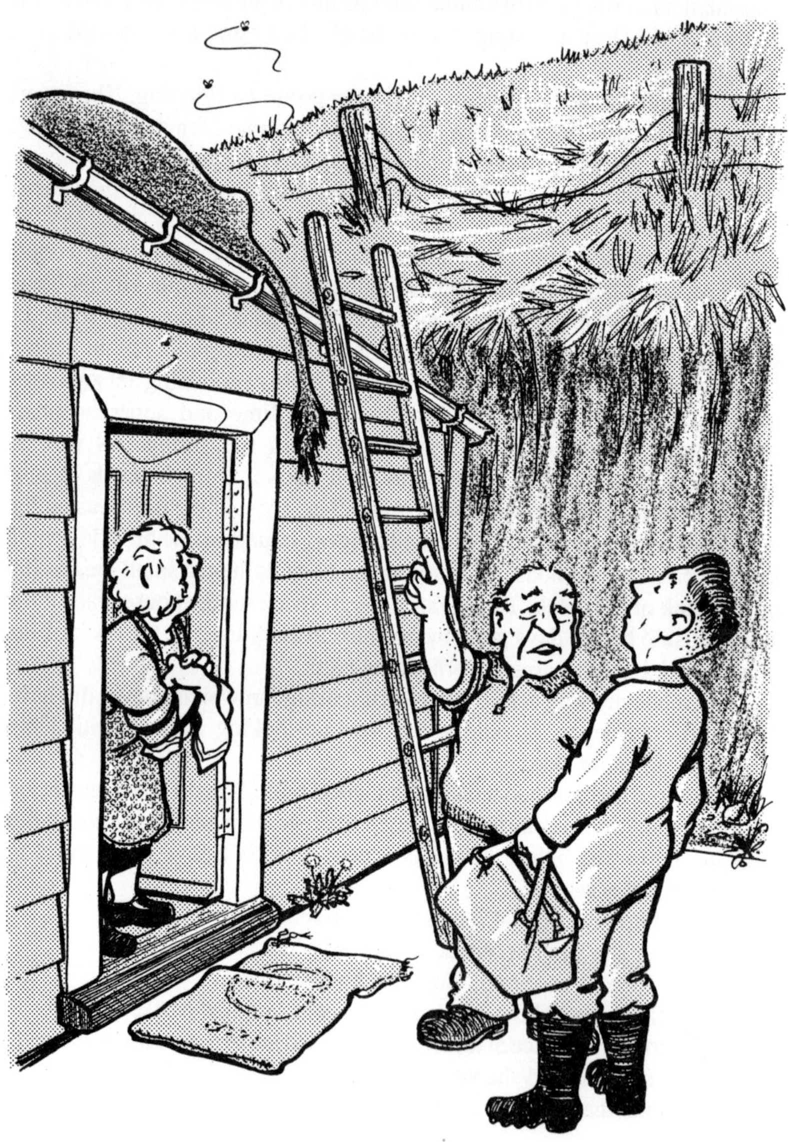

'We heard a bit of a bang and a crash in the dark just before we got up to milk,' continued Mick. ' I went outside to see what it was, but it was too dark and drizzling a bit as well — couldn't make it out meself although the sister's got a few ideas about things like that that happen at night! When we came in after milking we saw Rosie's tail hanging over the spouting above the kitchen door.'

I changed direction and soon saw a ladder propped against the wall of the kitchen. A bovine tail was indeed protruding from the roof above. As I cautiously ascended, the tail switched to and fro. I peered over the spouting and sure enough, on the roof lay a cow, flat out and showing all the signs of milk fever, but not yet at what I considered a critical stage.

'There doesn't seem to be a lot of point in treating her up there,' I said, descending to ground level, 'until we have thought of a way of getting her down.'

'Sure, and I've thought of that as well,' Mick assured me. 'If I stack a lot of hay bales on a slope like, we can just roll her off the roof and she'll come down just a treat.'

My experience of getting cows off roofs was a bit limited but I could see that Mick's plan might just work so I gave it provisional endorsement. At that point a tractor pulling a trailer roared over the hill and down the track to join us. There was apparently some sort of access to the farm by way of the plateau above. The tractor was driven by a bearded man who, despite the cool temperature, wore only a blue singlet and dirty shorts. On his feet were muddy gumboots. Pat, whose name also hinted at Irish ancestry, bid me the time of day and soon had the trailer of the tractor backed into Mick's hayshed. He, Mick, and to a lesser extent myself, soon had a full load of hay bales on the trailer. Within ten minutes the load was stacked against the kitchen wall, forming the beginnings of a ramp. The process was repeated and by then enough bales were in place as to reach just below the spouting. Hopefully it would provide a soft landing to Mother Earth for Rosie.

Pat and Mick climbed on to the roof and with each lifting one extremity, Rosie was encouraged to roll off the roof on to the ramp. She rolled once more, and ended up on the ground near where I stood. The wonder drug, calcium, soon returned her to a more alert state and we left her in a sitting position while we made our way into the kitchen where Sarah had laid on tea and scones.

I was about to take my leave when a bovine head appeared round the open kitchen door and, as cows have been known to do, emitted a 'moo...' which seemed to demand attention.

'Well, I'll be blowed!' exclaimed an astounded Pat. 'It's close on a miracle to be sure.'

'Rosie has a real hankering after a scone with a bit of jam on it,' explained Sarah. 'I expect she's a bit peckish after being up on the roof like all that time.'

Rosie showed her appreciation by accepting the offering with another moo before backing out of the kitchen door into her more usual environment.

'That's something else I've never seen before,' commented Pat as we thanked Sarah for her hospitality and went about our business.

This first so-called busy season was in fact not excessively so. Farmers, being by nature a cautious lot, were not over-anxious to employ the services of the unknown. They were also not overly keen to observe biological phenomena such as calving cows after dark. Therefore I was spared requests for many calls late in the day.

And so there was time for some relaxation when the work of the day was done. I recall with pleasure the weekly Saturday night visits to the crowded cinema in nearby Kaikohe. I remember His Worship the Mayor, Mr Guy, accompanied by Her Ladyship, almost regally descending the aisle towards their routinely reserved seats in the front row. They always arrived five minutes before the programme was due to start, and the patrons all reverently stood aside to let them pass. This formality completed, the raucous squawk of the kookaburra launched *Movietone News of Australia* and the programme began.

On these occasions I was often accompanied by George Pattison, a soldier in the Highland Light Infantry during the war. He had arrived in New Zealand to seek his fortune and join his sister Mrs Anderson, who was my part-time landlady. George was a welcome companion and was also a first-class table tennis player. Sometimes he partnered me on Tuesday nights, when I could get away, to play in the Ohaeawai Hall. The hall was continually in use for weddings, dairy company and other meetings, cinema shows, badminton and table tennis.

While the local band did not generate quite the same number of decibels as today's stereophonic apparatus, it did its best on dance nights and its output could be heard in the still of the night over quite a large area.

And so 1948 moved on its way. Having set in motion some improvements to my house I turned my attention to the grounds, all two acres of them. Firstly there was the footpath which was clearly inadequate for a busy vet needing to restock his car at regular intervals with supplies of medicines and other tools of trade. There was also the problem of the creek, identified by sound alone beneath its flourishing canopy of willow, bamboo and the rest.

Aggressive and positive action was called for. This was forthcoming through a yellow Caterpillar bulldozer of American origin equipped with winches front and rear, and driven by its owner, Pat McHugh. Pat soon had the willows and bamboo out of their watery bed and stacked on the rocky bank. In the warmer weather ahead, the impressive heap of vegetation became dry enough to burn. But the twigs and roots left behind soon sprang to life and in such a favourable environment created an ongoing problem.

The bulldozer also knocked down part of the road fence and made a track of sorts from road to dwelling. Because it was not metalled just then, and with the land sloping from road to house, it proved a lot easier for a car to get in than out. This problem was partially solved by establishing a number of alternative exits. If one didn't work you could always reverse the spinning wheels and try another!

One very necessary technical assistant to the busy season was the telephone. When I started work there nearly all the rural telephones in the north operated on the principle of the 'party line'. Residences, farms or even commercial properties, were linked by one telephone line to each other and the exchange. Each subscriber was allotted a letter which followed the number of the line; both number and letter had to be given by a caller wishing to communicate with a particular subscriber and each letter had a ring code allotted to it. If, for instance, on line number 25 subscriber A was sought, two long and one short rings were emitted. If subscriber D was needed the rings might be two short and one long.

All this sounds pretty complicated, but I must say that subscribers became quite adept at identifying and transmitting their own particular ring and rejecting others. It was also possible for subscribers on the same line to ring through to each other without reference to the central exchange. This was at no cost, so farmers and perhaps more often their wives, were able to chat with neighbours and friends close by. But when the line was so monopolised it was not possible for other subscribers to use it, this sometimes caused some rural mutterings. When a heavy user like myself was inserted into the party line system, as was the case when I boarded with the Baldwins, difficulties were common. The social function of the line was under pressure by what was, after all, a commercial undertaking. Social conversations sometimes effectively shut out receipt of a message about some ailing beast needing urgent attention. These problems were finally overcome when I had a private line installed at extra cost, linking my house directly to the exchange with none between.

The telephones of these times were community affairs and if privacy was sometimes at risk there was also a built-in information system which modern technology has yet to better. The Ohaeawai exchange was housed in an annex to the post office, strategically placed at the T-junction where Highway 1 turns sharply to the north and the bar of the 'T' continues towards Kaikohe and points west.

The window of the exchange was close to the switchboard and was usually open winter and summer. The operator had a clear view of the hotel across the road and the general store. As the store, the hotel and the post office formed a triangle, the operators had a visual map of much of what was happening. This they supplemented with titbits of the spoken word accidentally overheard while operating the manual switchboard.

On one occasion I was attempting in vain to reach a farmer client to fix a time for the vaccination of his stock. I was interrupted by the operator who told me that the family was off to Whangarei for the day to do some Christmas shopping. They had just passed the telephone exchange ten minutes before. Another time I was informed that a new baby had arrived during the night. The proud father, who had delivered his labouring wife to the maternity annex at Kawakawa in the wee small hours, had just left to inspect his new son who weighed seven pounds and eight ounces and was to be called Sam after his paternal grandfather — a fund of information at no extra charge!

Despite the vigilance and expertise of the girls in the telephone exchange and the dedication of the lady in the transport office, the receipt of messages was by no means an easy task. Calls outside office hours and at weekends were a special problem as I moved between Andersons' and my new house. When I was away on a call there was nobody around to record calls. Even when at home the telephone was hard to hear. Clients were on the whole pretty tolerant — more so then those would have been in longer established practices.

One dissatisfied farmer did take time off to express his displeasure in a letter to the board: 'Neglect of duty by a paid vet is not my idea of farming,' asserted the scribe.

'Nor mine either,' I hastened to assure the board.

The message had apparently originally been directed to the transport office from which the office lady was temporarily absent. The call was taken by one of the managers who, looking out of the window, saw me disappear into the store across the road. He did not record the message in the book provided but instead rang the store and conveyed it to one of the ladies who worked there. However, I had only wanted to buy some cigarettes and by the time the lady who had received the message had returned to the counter to deliver it, I had already gone. The message fell into a sort of communications vacuum from where it evoked no response. Such was life, and I could see that my skin would have to grow a bit thicker if I was going to last the pace.

I noticed early on that the pattern of animal disease in New Zealand was less complex than in Britain, Europe and some of the tropical countries I had visited. Conditions like anthrax, rinderpest, rabies, foreign bodies in the stomach impinging on the heart, and scrapie in sheep were absent or seldom occurred.

One condition which was common in New Zealand was mastitis or, as local farmers called, mammitis. This was an inflammation of the bovine udder. The vulnerability of udder to various infections had been brought about by the selective breeding of the dairy cow to ensure that she produced as much milk as possible. For that purpose a very large udder was necessary. Because it was so big and so pendulous it became susceptible to traumatic damage and infection. I was involved at one time in the supervision of a number of government owned dairy herds in India and the incidence of mastitis there was very low — but there, individual cow production was measured in pints rather than gallons.

In New Zealand the disease, most likely the most common human or animal bacterial infection around, has defied control for many years. A variety of germs can be involved and it is thought that most infections are introduced through the teats particularly at the time of milking. This is when the hands of milkers, cups of milking machines, and various cloths and other equipment are eagerly seized upon by bacteria as vehicles to facilitate their nefarious propagation. Cups left milking when there is no more milk left to withdraw, and machines producing a vacuum pressure higher than necessary, could cause bruising and bleeding of sensitive tissues. This provided a mixture of blood and milk — an ideal medium in which bacteria could prosper.

Even in cows which had apparently recovered, infection tended to continue to lurk in the maze of ducts and honeycomb of glands which make up the udder. Conditions such as the stress of calving, cold or heat, underfeeding or injury, could cause the mastitis to blossom and cause untold problems.

It was mastitis which caused me the most thought for I felt relatively powerless in dealing with it. The age of antibiotics had still to come and when it did, that caused its own special problems. Meantime, in acute cases, heavy doses of sulphanilamide sometimes saved a life if not an udder. Injection into the udder of derivatives of a yellow dye called acriflavine was recommended, but I found it had a limited benefit. The colour of the stuff stained anything with which it came in contact bright yellow. Its only use appeared to be as a placebo for the owner if not the patient!

Mud was again a factor which encouraged the survival of the causal organism. It provided moisture and relative warmth which was ideal for bacterial survival. If the cocktail was completed by the addition of a little milk from time to time, there was multiplication as well.

Speaking of mud, by now it was mid-November and the sun was high in the sky and quite hot. I had been called to attend a cow suffering from mastitis and the patient had been shut in the cowyard and exposed to the heat of the sun. I found the udder encased in a jacket of what looked and felt like concrete. In fact it was a thick coating of mud, baked hard by the sun. I needed a hammer to crack the jacket and remove it for the examination.

All this, I suppose, sounds pretty grim stuff. I should point out that the lot of the dairy cow in those times was not always a happy one. At the risk of confounding those who regard the country life as always idyllic I am placing some of its shortcomings on record.

Another creature often disadvantaged was the pig. Very large amounts of bacon and pork must have been consumed in the fifties because nearly every dairy farmer kept some pigs. They were used as a means of disposing of the very great amount of skim milk left over after the cream was separated. Many pigs were fed on a diet of skim milk alone. Coupled with the poor conditions under which they were kept, they were predisposed to enteric diseases of the salmonella group. This killed off pigs in fairly large numbers.

Pig houses were, at best, often basic buildings of wood or corrugated iron. They were too cold in winter and too hot in summer. The unpaved pens often became mudbaths when it rained, which was often. This was appreciated by wallowing porcines on the one hand but on the other when mixed with a bit of 'skim dick' (as the skimmed milk was popularly called) was perfect for bacterial survival and multiplication. Another condition which was a result of the primitive management conditions was called necrotic ulcer — a circular spreading ulcer spreading on the face, jaw and other places. Until controlled by penicillin, this was a serious problem which caused much suffering and concern.

The breeding sows most likely had the best of it, at least until they had their litters. The idea was to have the sows farrowing about the same time as the cows started to calve. Before then there was no milk so the practice was to allow the sows free range on the farm with grass as the only staple diet plus anything else they could pick up. Sows were usually good mothers and took care to farrow in places as sheltered as possible.

I recall the case of one client who had purchased a bull at a sale somewhere down south. As was often the case, he took delivery of the animal late at night when the weather was wet as well as stormy. The truck driver didn't need too much persuasion to stay the night and after unloading the bull was anxious to escape to the warmth of the farm kitchen. In his haste he neglected to fasten the tailboard of his truck which had been used as a ramp to unload the bull. Next morning he hastened on his way after securing it, but because it was still dark he failed to look inside. On arrival at his home base on the other side of Auckland he opened the back to find a sow with a litter of seven enjoying the

comfort of the straw bed provided for the safe transport of my client's bull.
The sow's owner was also more than a little surprised when he received a
telephone call inquiring if he had missed a sow and, if so, if he had any
suggestions as to how the itinerant pig might be returned. I guess they worked
something out!

Some farmers though, were very successful with their pigs. They
provided a variation and supplement to the skim milk diet through growing
maize, sugar beet and other crops, as well as purchasing meat meal and barley
meal. These were greatly appreciated by the fast-growing porkers.
Investment in a properly constructed piggery always paid off as the pig is a
creature very susceptible to extremes of temperature, especially cold
draughts. It may have been a coincidence, but I noticed that the most
successful pig farmers among my clients appeared to have Irish names or had
their origins in that country. It was an indication perhaps that ways with
animals, as indeed other things, may be something inherited from long ago.

The Vet Takes a Wife

Come November, things eased off and I was able to give some time again to the grounds of the house. Under the influence of a wet and warm spring they were showing their true potential. This was particularly true of the creek bed where bamboo and willow, unabashed by the assault of the bulldozer only a few weeks before, were doing their best to retaliate. They had established aggressive shoots which, if left alone, would clearly have resulted in a jungle more dense than before. I sought advice from some of my clients and they told me that a chemical called sodium chlorate in spray form might be effective. I acquired some of the stuff and attacked the growth with as much vigour as I could muster, resulting in a temporary browning off of the vegetation and some pain in a few muscles I didn't previously know I had. I later discovered more powerful chemicals, which together with nibbling sheep eventually managed to rid the creek of its weeds and establish the first stage of what many years later was to become quite a showplace.

We celebrated Guy Fawkes day in style with a few friends and a crate of beer, and set alight the big heap of rubbish dragged out by the bulldozer which I had back. Pat McHugh had created a smooth track over the now dried out soil, extending it into a circular turn around in front of the house. I had several trucks of red scoria brought in from a nearby volcanic quarry and when that had settled in, more loads of river shingle from a creek behind Eric Walker's house at Pakaraka. The luxury of all-weather access was in place at last.

Inside my contractors of various ages, trades and dispositions proceeded as inclination and availability of materials took them. The smell of newly sawn timber, or freshly applied paint or varnish was a source of encouragement as well as a measure of progress.

But changes were afoot and important steps imminent. I had arranged to take two weeks annual leave early in January when wedding bells would toll and the newlyweds would honeymoon in Australia.

Meanwhile, I was concerned about my car which had survived the busy season — but only just. The car wasn't up to the roads of crushed rock or being pushed or pulled by man or horse or tractor or grader when it was forced to surrender to the environment. The wedding ceremony was scheduled to take place some way south and while it was the bride's privilege to be a trifle late at church on the day, I wondered if in our case it might be the bridegroom. I had visions of being stranded by the roadside somewhere, causing consternation among those assembled by my failure to arrive.

I promptly consulted my mechanics who had performed remarkable feats of engineering to keep me on the road. They believed that as the roads on which I would be travelling would be of a higher standard than those of the rural mid-north, I would have a 50-50 chance of reaching my objective.

I had the springs set up and the unreliable brakes adjusted for the fifth time in as many months. There was also the odd bit of welding carried out before removing a few pounds of desiccated mud from the floor and what looked to be nearly as much dust from the upholstery and roof lining. The original blue finish had become quite pale but a couple of hours with a duster and some polish restored something of a sheen. And so it was, that having received an assurance from painter Teddy Jones and poker-faced plumber Eric Walker that all would be well on my return, I took my leave of Ohaeawai to embark on a venture as different as it was new.

The trip to Auckland at that time was not one to be undertaken lightly. The road as far as Whangarei was largely metalled and with a fair number of buses, cars, cream trucks, petrol tankers, herds of cows and flocks of sheep the trip could be quite exciting. Beyond Whangarei there was a fair proportion of sealed highway and better progress could be made until the Waitemata Harbour loomed ahead. This sea barrier had to be crossed by ferry unless a much longer detour to the west was taken. The ferries proceeded from either Devonport or Northcote and there was usually a waiting time, which at weekends or on holidays could be a fair while. The trip from the Bay of Islands to Queen Street could take all of five hours.

My wedding was of interest in that no guests came from my side of the family. The 12,000 miles of land and water between myself and the land of my fathers proved an effective barrier, although we had many messages of goodwill. This meant that all the guests present, and there seemed to be plenty of them, were more or less acquainted with each other and this made for a day of reunion as well as celebration.

The next day we were passengers to Sydney in a DC6 aircraft rising into the skies above Whenuapai. We spent the next 10 days touring the eastern seaboard before returning to Auckland's Mechanics Bay in the flying boat *Australia 2*.

Travel by flying boat was slow but relaxing. I guess one reason was the thought that although there was a lot of water below, we were travelling in what was as much a boat as an aeroplane. If we had to come down we would float, although for how long I did not know. The other reason was that there was lots of room inside. One could wander about at will and chat with others while admiring the cloudscape around and above and the seascape below. Facilities such as those routinely provided in the flying boats are nowadays available only to the rich who can afford a first-class ticket in jumbo jets.

Auckland always seemed to me a bit dowdy and colonial after journeys overseas, particularly if you arrived at the weekend. However, Australia in 1949 left me with the impression of having big, fast moving cities with a lot of nothing in-between. The places we stayed at between the cities were, I thought, fairly primitive.

New Zealand on the other hand had cities of more modest proportion and outlook, with less of a void in-between. But as we found on the homeward trail, planning and ingenuity were needed to acquire even a cup of tea and a sandwich in the rural north.

I speak only in a material sense because in New Zealand there is something of interest around every corner, be it green farmland with animals grazing, limpid lake or rushing river, or the coastline of beautiful beach or sentinel rocks on which the mighty ocean finally surrenders its claim to the land in clouds of spray.

It was dark when we arrived home and it took me some time to find where Jack Ireland had hidden the key. A touch of a switch and a flood of light revealed all. I can't help but reiterate what a difference a bit of paint and paper can make. The tradesmen, conscious of our imminent arrival had performed nobly and had been at pains to tidy up the place a bit. There was even a bunch of flowers in a jam jar on the Chinese table with its bamboo legs. We were both quite impressed. I suppose that gaining a house, a wife, a car and a practice, even if I didn't own it, within a year of arrival in the promised land was progress. However, it left the achiever in me still champing at the bit.

Some oak furniture had been ordered from Auckland and in our absence this had been delivered and stacked on the veranda. Luckily it had not rained. My first task was to assemble beds and put the new dressing-table in place against the wall in what we called the master bedroom, for all the bedrooms were about the same size.

The next day it was back to work and I made the first move in my animal disease control programme. I drafted a circular to suppliers of both dairy companies inviting them to present their current crop of heifer calves for vaccination against brucellosis or contagious abortion. The calves needed to be vaccinated between the age of six and eight months which meant that the programme was already late. But it was better late than never. It was going to be a couple of years before the first vaccinated calves would be ready to have their own calves and the benefit of the protective inoculation would be revealed.

The vaccine had to be obtained from the Commonwealth Serum Laboratory in Australia and this caused further delay although I had taken the precaution of ordering some in advance. This supply arrived within a week and clients' requests for the service began to build. The programme was in place.

I had always regarded my car with something of the affection usually reserved for an aging relative or a well-loved pet. Although it had responded nobly to the various long trips associated with our nuptial celebrations, I felt that I could be chancing my arm to hold on to it for much longer. In addition, my wife liked to drive sometimes and the pressure needed to operate the braking system was too much for her to generate.

We therefore headed south again to see what we could find. Near Wellsford the sun completely dazzled the driver of a car heading north who swung round a bend over to our side of the road. The scrub again proved to be a refuge and perhaps life-saver. Thankfully very much alive we arrived in Auckland and I had the chance of introducing my wife to the delights of the Star Hotel.

Next day we were afoot early, ready to do business or combat with the car dealers of Auckland. I had been warned that dealing with these gentlemen could, on occasions, be unrewarding as well as unprofitable. However, cars such as mine were well suited to the city environment and it was still of fairly recent vintage. Its turbulent past was largely discounted and I managed to obtain a satisfactory trade-in price. In fact it was better than what I had hoped for.

My new vehicle was a 1939 V-8 coupe, a car much older but far tougher than my previous one. I was assured it was ideal for the roads and other places over which I had to travel. The new car, if it could be so called, was the colour of bleached sand and stood me in good stead for several years. Eventually it hit a rock in Chappie Baldwin's paddock, damaging the front axle. Thereafter it needed periodic unbending to keep the wheels in alignment as they had developed a tendency to splay, leading to uneven tyre wear. However, its purchase was a step in the right direction. Propelled by the powerful V-8 motor, we returned north in a fashion much faster than that in which we had come.

Early Hazards and Hopes

By the time we reached home, more vaccine had arrived and another 20 or more farmers had indicated their willingness to have their calves vaccinated. Among the applications was one in which a farmer had scribbled on the back that such matters were best left for nature to take its course. That was exactly what nature had been doing. Nature does not always support that which man decrees. By now around 4,000 calves were destined to receive protective inoculation against the ravages of brucellosis. This took a bit of organisation. Clearly it was best to carry out the operation on a geographical basis with about a dozen properties visited each day. I wondered what sort of cooperation would be my lot, but I found that by ringing two or three nights before, nearly all farmers were able and willing to have their calves assembled at the time advised. This was extremely important. If even one farmer was late in yarding his calves, especially early in the day, the lapse had a domino effect which delayed the programme and tended to interfere with afternoon milking — a cardinal sin.

The conditions under which the calves were assembled was another matter. This was something new for most farmers who had never been so involved before. Many were uncertain as to what was required. Calves were left loose in the cowshed, jammed in milking bails, in races with impossibly high sides, in races meant for sheep with sides so low that apprehensive calves could escape with ease and disappear with tails high in the air across the paddock. I recall one mob crushed in a corner behind an old bedstead. Altogether it proved to be a bit of a circus, with farmers, together with their dogs and calves, the clowns and myself the ringmaster.

All this, despite the delays, would have had its funny side apart from one thing. The milky white vaccine from Australia, dispensed in 100cc bottles with a rubber cap, looked innocuous enough, but here was a tiger by the tail — a tail my clients and myself were about to unwittingly grasp. The slightest prick from the needle impregnated with vaccine was enough to initiate the severe undulant fever in people. With calves unused to restraint and confined in inadequate ways, and owners often clad in minimal clothing leaving large areas of target skin exposed, the risk of accidental inoculation of unsuspecting clients was a real one. It concerned me for many years to come.

My own left hand which I used to raise a tent of skin on the neck of the patient, was very vulnerable. There was another problem. Syringes of the day had not been adapted for mass vaccination. The best I could find was an Australian model which carried only five doses when fully loaded. It needed to be refilled after five calves were vaccinated. After a few punctures the rubber cap on the vaccine bottle tended to become pervious with the result that, from time to time, some leakage of the deadly stuff took place, dribbling down the side of the syringe on to the hand of the operator; in this case me. Changes in pressure could also spray vaccine in directions it was not supposed to go, like human eyes. If this happened, undulant fever could follow or there could be a severe local reaction to the vaccine. This could result in permanent damage to the eyes or other part of the body.

The calves however, despite receiving a full 5 c.c. dose, appeared to suffer no serious problems apart from being a bit off-colour for a day or two. As time went by I became a lot more conscious of the dangers inherent in the use of this vaccine and wore a heavy leather gauntlet on my left hand while in action. Automatic multiple vaccinators were later available, which called for but one puncture of the bottle's seal thus minimising leakage and the use of pressure-driven dangerous aerosols. But all this was still to come.

Meanwhile, the luck of my clients and myself held, at least until the penultimate batch of calves for the season was yarded for my attention. Paradoxically, the race was one of the better ones — a high sheep drafting race allowing good access to the calves' neck. The fourth calf must have sensed that something unpleasant was about to happen and maybe the needle I was using had lost its edge. Just as a blunt knife is most likely to cut its user, the extra pressure needed to cause a blunt needle to penetrate can, if misdirected, guide the needle to places not intended. As I jabbed, the calf jumped. The needle, glancing, off at a tangent, penetrated my left hand just where the thumb joins the rest of it. I hastily poured on some disinfectant and hoped for the best.

Nothing much happened for a couple of days and with a degree of thankfulness I completed my vaccination programme. It was birthday time for us and this was another cause for celebration. My punctured hand had been fairly peaceful but now the redness, heat and pain of an acute inflammatory process became apparent. At the same time a gloomy malaise descended on the vet, making life less than interesting. A visit to the physician, armed with an empty vaccine bottle as evidence, didn't tax his diagnostic skill too much but the patient looked bad enough to suggest a visit to the hospital for a few tests and the like.

'Most interesting,' pronounced the Superintendent at the hospital and went off to read up his books on the subject. I was consigned to a private room, a privilege I later discovered was for the distinguished, or for those whose prognosis was a little on the gloomy side. Treatment, it was decided, should be the best available even if it bore little relationship to the disease from which I now suffered. Fairly toxic sulphadiazine six hourly, penicillin and streptomycin by injection four hourly, plus a few poultices and antipyretics were prescribed. I hadn't felt so perforated since having a course of 14 injections after handling a rabid dog in India some four years before.

Blood samples were despatched to Dunedin to see what could be made of the problem. Someone said that when the titre in my blood started to fall things would be better, but until then fingers would need to be kept crossed. As I knew that the titre might be expected to rise for quite a while I detected something of a hole in this argument. But it was a lot easier to get into hospital than escape from it, and meantime the onslaught of chemotherapy, orally and parentally, continued. Thankfully I survived the treatment.

To sustain me were daily visits from my wife, and occasional ones from others who brought books and grapes and sometimes seemed to think that a vet getting in the way of a needle intended for his patient was a bit of a joke. After five weeks my titre began to fall. The hospital was jubilant at having effected a cure, although a bit sad I thought at having to lose its longest lasting inmate in the men's ward, and such an interesting one at that!

Back in circulation, two stone lighter and a bit wiser, it took a while to find my land legs again. It was just as well that the practice was not making too many demands on me, in a physical sense at least. All this may have been something of a blessing in disguise because I have no doubt that by the time I left hospital my immunity to brucellosis had climbed to a high level, even if it had been earned the hard way. I was thus protected from subsequent natural infection from stock, as well as further accidental prods from vaccine-bearing needles.

It was around this time that the few vets in the north decided to form an association and to seek affiliation with the parent New Zealand Veterinary Association headquartered in Hamilton, around which most of the practising vets in New Zealand were then located. The government vet in Whangarei was Douglas Munro Corbett, a Scot of short stature and forthright manner and with whom I retain a pleasing acquaintance to this day. He acted as liaison, while Geoff Moon from Warkworth, John McDonald from Ruawai, a rather mysterious colleague from Dargaville, and a Pole called Ropert, became foundation members. Geoff later became a bird photographer of international acclaim. I do not recall if I was the foundation president or became president soon after.

The branch had regular meetings each month in Whangarei. As numbers grew, activities and the breadth of topic and discussion widened with experts from veterinary and related fields invited to address us. Remits were formulated for consideration by the national body or its council.

The veterinary profession in New Zealand was now in a very positive evolutionary stage as post-war graduates from Sydney took up appointments, supplemented by graduates mainly from Britain. A new identity was being established, which although in no way competent to cope with the powerful farming lobby and similar edifices of influence, was at least in being. The annual conferences in the fifties were usually held late January at the Chateau Tongariro. As the profession at this time was in its youth the same applied to its members and some of the conferences were fairly wild affairs. It was just as well they were held at National Park, well away from any centre of population where people might have thought the night was time to sleep.

Most vets arrived at the Chateau by road, but I recall on one occasion surveying the misty, drizzly landscape from my bedroom window and detecting the roar of a still invisible low-flying aircraft. A single-engined machine emerged from the gloom, passed a few feet above where I stood, and made a safe but rather erratic landing on the golf course below. From the cabin door there emerged two white-faced vets who had been persuaded to join the aircraft at Wanganui, en route from its home base in the South Island. The pilot, also a vet, appeared unperturbed, although one of his colleagues who also held a pilot's licence, later told me that this particular aviator would often fly when the birds were grounded! I think his passengers went home by bus.

Although much of the activity at these conferences was social and often of a fairly vigorous nature, many important issues were discussed and no doubt had an impact on significant events yet to happen. The establishment of a veterinary school was one topic which was regularly discussed. New Zealand, despite having a very large animal population on which its economy almost entirely depended, had curiously neglected to establish such a school.

The need for a scheme to eradicate bovine tuberculosis was constantly brought to the attention of government and farmers' organisations. Criticism of the club system of practice was also much to the fore at these conferences. There was clearly an underlying discontent but the new graduate, who at that time constituted the majority, had neither the means nor the confidence to jump over the wall into the unknown shadows of private enterprise. I think that this was a mistake, for it meant a continuing domination of the practicing profession by its farmer clients, a situation which was to continue for some time yet.

Returning to the practice at home there was one service industry to which

I logically should make reference. When I started there was little interest in the supply of veterinary medicines. The local chemist did some low-profile business and the many stock firms also supplied various drenches and other items, often with inadequate advice as to how these should be used. But all this was about to change for a number of reasons. In the first place many of the newly available so-called ethical drugs, like the sulphas and antibiotics, were available only through a registered veterinary surgeon. These drugs were remarkably effective in the treatment of a number of common stock ailments. When farmers became aware of this, the business boomed and soon justified the employment of a number of salespeople by various firms anxious to bring their wares to the attention of the practicing profession.

Many of these 'reps' as they were called, worked hard and were people of personality. However, most of my colleagues and myself did not always welcome their presence, chiefly because they always seemed to have time to talk and we did not. It was no joy after dashing back at the end of a busy morning, hoping for a quick lunch before embarking on an even busier afternoon, to find a couple of travellers parked in the drive vying for my time in competition with, perhaps, a lady with a sick cat in a carton and a man nursing a pet dog with a broken leg.

Nonetheless, I used to enjoy discussion with these reps in the old surgery behind the house. They often brought news of, and messages from colleagues with whom I had too little contact. They also recounted the latest advances in the veterinary pharmaceutical field with, of course, understandable bias towards the product they were promoting. Some were even quick to offer their services as erstwhile assistants if imminent surgery called for restraint of a patient. I recall once having to temporarily abandon my patient to administer first aid to one young rep. His enthusiasm to assist far exceeded his capacity to survive the sight of blood flowing from within the peritoneal cavity of an anaesthetised poodle. The dog was secured to the operating table ready to lose a large but benign growth flourishing on one of her more vital organs.

There is also the story of a young lady – the only female rep I had thus far encountered — who worked for a firm specialising in the sale of veterinary instruments. On this occasion she was demonstrating the use of a prodder made in Germany. This useful machine generated an electric charge by way of a manually operated lever. It was sufficiently powerful enough to encourage a cow, recumbent for psychological rather than strictly veterinary reasons, to try to get to her feet. This was an important step towards recovery, especially in the wet and cold of winter. As a further advertisement for the effectiveness of the prodder she told me that when up north she always took one to bed with her and found it the ideal means to repel any of the locals bent on the invasion of her privacy. Initiative and versatility indeed, but no advertisement for where we lived!

As I regained some strength after the brucellosis incident, we were able again to turn our attention to the house. We decided the front veranda would have to go as it really was beyond repair. The spectre of clients disappearing through its floor was continually with us. This was a pity for, to some extent it destroyed the character of the house. But once the decision had been made I attacked it with axe, crowbar and newly-found vigour. Soon an imposing heap of kauri firewood raised itself at the back of the house while the front assumed a rather flat denuded appearance, with the incongruous strips of unpainted weatherboard indicating where the veranda had once been attached.

With the expertise of local carpenter Bill Woods, we created a new entry way in the front, featuring the attractive old kauri door recovered from its original position at the end of the passage. A couple of new windows on either side of the door and three new concrete steps leading up to the entrance completed the transformation. The front door wasn't used all that often but the aesthetic impact was, we thought, pleasing.

While the carpenter was on the job we decided that we could just afford a new garage sheathed in weatherboard and floored in concrete, built just outside the back door. As a lean-to and an afterthought there emerged a fowl house leading to a hastily constructed netting-enclosed run within which flourished an abundance of kikuyu grass and a prolific plum tree. A chook house without chooks wasn't much of a game so we bought about a dozen Rhode Island Red pullets and were soon self-supporting in eggs — brown ones which we liked.

Eggs were now no problem but milk was. I solved this by purchasing a newly-calved Shorthorn heifer, complete with calf, for £17 from a farm at Waimate North. It was not possible for us to milk this acquisition ourselves but I managed to persuade Eric Baldwin, until lately my landlord and saviour in many respects, to sharemilk her with us. We got our daily milk from his shed and he got the balance and the calf. Somehow, the Department of Agriculture became aware of this satisfactory arrangement and informed my supplier that as his cowshed was not registered within the town milk system he would have to stop supplying us. This created something of a crisis, for at that time there was no shop or dairy in the township which sold milk. Residents mainly relied on the production from house cows grazing in nearby paddocks and milked by their individual or collective owners. Such animals were not milked through a cowshed and thus were apparently immune from the heavy hand of officialdom. I could not see a lot of difference in that system from the one we were using so I wrote a letter to the Minister of Agriculture explaining our milkless predicament. The answer, after all, was simple. A few sheets of painted hardboard nailed above the milk vat and Eric was awarded a temporary town milk licence. Wonders never cease! Ten years later the same shed, albeit much upgraded, was supplying town milk on a far greater scale — with myself as owner.

All the house alterations naturally needed to be followed up with some paint and as our funds were now at a cyclical low I resolved to tackle this job myself, despite my enthusiasm being well ahead of my experience. A ladder was the first necessity and I constructed one from some of the more-sound pieces of three by two from the demolished veranda. A number of gallon tins of 'roof red' paint was purchased from the North Auckland Farmer's Store in Kaikohe. I promptly found out what extraordinary strength of wrist and arm was needed to persuade the solid putty-like mass resting on the bottom of each tin to combine with the more liquid constitituents on top. Mixing took quite some time and was good training for the erstwhile painter, not only for his painting project, but for the calving season when muscular development of the wrists and arms was a useful asset. A supply of turpentine and brushes completed my armoury.

With an apprehensive wife supporting the swaying homemade ladder I clambered on to the roof bearing a wire brush, a few square feet of coarse sandpaper, several cans of paint, a bottle of turps and a couple of paint brushes. I didn't last too long though for I discovered the southern sun. It produced a temperature at which eggs and amateur painting vets could easily have fried. Protective clothing in the form of overalls was called for, and thus attired I made a second attempt.

The hot roof though, was good for painting and the oil-based paint flowed on with surprising ease and pleasing result. It took about a week, off and on, to complete the job and I found that the paint, eager to establish an effective bond with the iron roof, had a similar affinity with the exposed parts of myself. Efforts to remove the unwanted red spots were mostly in vain and I appeared as if I had been afflicted by some unusual exotic disease.

My clients, not slow to sum up the situation, made remarks like, 'Doin' some paintin' then — I see you got some on your face.'

This became a bit tiresome after a few repeats but was often followed by some helpful advice from authorities far more competent than myself and all this was to stand me in good stead when I tackled the walls and outbuildings. These proved to be far easier than the roof, and a lot cooler.

The place was looking pretty smart now but I was concerned about one thing. The path from back door to front, and then round the corner to the surgery, was still ill-defined but heavily used. I could see that when winter came, the volcanic soil would become wet and muddy with a fair proportion of this being transferred inside to the house or surgery. As always, Eric Baldwin was my willing aid and he arrived complete with concrete mixer and motor strapped to the luggage rack of his small car. I arranged for a load of shingle from the creek at Pakaraka to be delivered, together with a dozen bags of cement from the dairy factory and some red scoria from a nearby quarry for the foundation. We established a scoria base and it was not long before a concrete path extended around the house.

By now the leaves of autumn had fallen for the second time since I arrived in this new land. Autumn rains were turning pastures brown to pastures green, while the cows were becoming more placid and perceptibly more pregnant. With a diminished flow of milk they would mostly make their way to the milking sheds only once, rather than twice a day. Soon their milk was to cease altogether as their owners called it a day and sometimes took their holidays during the two months or so the cows remained out of production.

The new calving season was now upon me but this time it was different. The major miracle of calcium, and a few minor ones, were by now fairly common knowledge and from June the first the telephone was rarely silent. On Sundays the telephone exchange closed at eight and unless my clients could get in touch with me before that hour, short of a personal visit, there was no way that I could be easily contacted until six next morning. My clients were however quite well aware of this limitation so it was not unusual for the bell to demand attention in that last quarter-of-an-hour before the line went temporarily dead.

So it was one Sunday night in July. A voice which sounded far away informed me that a cow at Ivydale, on the shores of the Hokianga Harbour, had been trying to calve all day with no result. I suggested that an earlier call would have received more sympathetic attention from the vet and been more rewarding for the patient, but this attracted no comment. I never liked leaving calving cases longer than what was necessary.

'Where do you live?' I inquired.

'Well,' said my new client, 'it's a bit hard to explain, but tell you what, if you come up the road through Ivydale I'll come down to the gate and meet you by the cream stand; that way you won't be able to miss the place.'

I had to be satisfied with this rather tentative arrangement and set off into the night. The road as far as Okaihau wasn't all that bad but after that things got a bit rough. On the Utakura Hill I had a near miss when a couple of Herefords, grazing on the roadside, loomed within my headlights before retreating in confusion into the fern. A bit further on a horse jumped off a bank ahead and galloped off, throwing up a shower of metal which bombarded my windscreen. The startled equine gave up half-a-mile down the road and cleared the road fence into some paddock. Anticipating a rendezvous at

Ivydale, I slowed down, which was just as well. My client was not yet visible as the road became virtually two metalled strips separated by tufted grass in-between. Suddenly there was nothing but my headlights illuminating a void. I stood on the brakes and skidded to a standstill within a couple of feet from the edge of a cliff. Far below in the moonlight, I could just detect waves breaking on a rocky shore. It appeared that I had entered a quarry of some sort. Shaken by the near miss, I cautiously reversed the car from the edge of the abyss. It was then that I noticed an open gate mostly concealed by fern, to which a notice had been attached bearing the legend 'Private - No Entry'.

About a mile down the road in the reverse direction I spied a figure wearing a cowboy hat and a battledress blouse above waterproof leggings. He was leaning on a creamstand smoking a pipe, stoked with tobacco of a less expensive sort.

'You were quick,' remarked my client. 'I must have missed you.'

I informed the pipe-smoking farmer of my recent experience and he said that the jokers who owned the quarry should keep the gate shut or somebody would get killed.

'Like me,' I thought.

'Well,' I said, reaching the conclusion that further discussion about the dangerous quarry would not be profitable, 'how do we get to the cowshed?'

'It's like this,' said my client. 'In the summer you could drive up, no sweat, but just now it's too wet and all that rain we had last week washed out a culvert. Not to worry, I've got a horse here and he'll get you up there like one thing; it's only about a mile.'

On this discouraging note the farmer led not one, but two horses out of the shadow of the creamstand. I recovered some calving gear from the car and packed it in a hold-all hoping that I would need nothing more sophisticated. My client extinguished his pipe, grabbed my bag and mounted one of the horses, before galloping off into the moonlight. I clambered onto my steed, which like most New Zealand horses had a bit of thoroughbred in him. Feeling a competitive urge he pricked up his ears and dashed off in pursuit. My horse certainly knew the way and the trip, apart from an unexpected six-foot leap across the washed-out culvert, was exciting rather than especially dangerous.

In five minutes or so we approached the cowshed, dimly lit by a kerosene lantern. Electric power had not yet penetrated up this remote valley. On dismounting I found the farmer scratching his well-thatched head and looking at a gap in the ti-tree rails surrounding the yard of his cowshed.

'You know,' he said. 'This must be about the silliest thing I've ever done —she must have got out. She'll be in that totara bush somewhere but there's no show of finding her tonight. I tell you what, I'll get the dogs on to her in the morning and give you another ring.'

All this left me fairly speechless and I thought I'd better count ten before replying.

'You do that,' was all I could say.

I never did hear any more about that cow or her owner, which for them and certainly for me was maybe just as well.

I have mentioned before that many of the roads on which I had cause to travel left a lot to be desired and there is no doubt that this was one of my chief problems. Even Highway 1 was mostly metalled and heavy vehicles like buses (or service cars as they were then known), cream trucks and the like, threw the metal into unstable ridges sometimes all of a foot high. The tyres of lesser vehicles found it difficult to secure a hold, resulting in the cars quite often sliding sideways into the road verge. Luckily, this was usually fairly wide and covered in thick vegetation, acting as a cushion and preventing further disaster.

Another problem was one-way bridges or culverts—there were eight, for instance, between Ohaeawai and Kaikohe, a distance of only six miles. On minor roads these were encountered without warning and if another vehicle or wandering animal had claimed prior occupancy, good brakes and a cool head were needed for survival. A still further hazard was stock. In winter, when many farms were short of grass, it was common practice for stock to be turned out on to the roadside verges or the 'long acre' as it was called, where during the prolific months of summer there was significant growth of grass and other vegetation. It provided a welcome, if unofficial, reserve of winter feed. This idea is still with us, but nowadays the use of the electric fence enables the verges to be grazed without stock creating a traffic hazard.

Black cattle were a particular hazard in the dark with only their shining eyes being visible, and then only if the beam of headlights were directed straight at the 'target', for that is what they too often turned out to be. Horses were also a special danger, for in the days of which I write, large numbers of apparently ownerless equines survived in the bush or on poorly fenced farms. A fair proportion of these used to find their way onto the roads. Because they were usually dark-coloured and difficult to see they were a definite menace. They also had a tendency to jump off banks when disturbed, sometimes landing on top of vehicles passing below. None landed atop my vehicles although I had a few near misses. The long established Ohaeawai taxi driver was less fortunate for he told me that his car had been bestridden by flying equines on three occasions, each time inflicting significant damage from which the local panelbeater profited. Periodic efforts were made by the Ministry of Transport to find owners of these horses but with limited success. One drive netted several hundred which were ultimately slaughtered at the

Moerewa works, a practice later prohibited because our American customers feared that horse meat might in some way be substituted for the beef they wanted and paid for.

As the busy season progressed I discovered that the district was host to another disease which I, nor anyone else, had identified around here before. The most dramatic episode I encountered occurred on Christmas morning when Charlie Mason, our neighbour from just across the road, interrupted our festive mood. Appearing on the doorstep he told me that he had found three of his eight calves dead as he was returning home after morning milking.

It didn't take me long to cross the road and, sure enough, three big, well-conditioned Jersey calves lay stretched out on the banks of a stream. Nearby was Charlie's impressive two-storeyed house called appropriately *Paheke*, built in 1865 on the banks of a small stream and of historical significance. On approaching one of the casualties I noticed some blood-stained froth at the nose and swelling around the uppermost hip. When I tentatively pressed this swelling with a forefinger it squelched. When I made a small incision into its depths some gas escaped and the muscle mass below the skin had the appearance of black mince, interspersed with bubbles of gas. A rancid smell drifted here and there on the westerly zephyrs — putrefaction had clearly set in although the calf could only have been dead hours at the most.

'I think you have a problem in the way of Blackleg,' I told Charlie, and a neighbour who with hands on hips had been peering over my shoulder.

'And what,' inquired Charlie, never the easiest one in the world to convince, 'may that be?'

'It's caused by a germ of the clostridial, anaerobic group,' I said, using terms which later experience taught me to simplify when talking to clients. 'It normally lives a peaceful life in what is called spore form, enclosed in a hard tough shell — a bit like a coconut but so small it can't be seen without a microscope. Now this spore can survive the toughest of conditions and can even be boiled for a while without doing it too much damage; it is highly transportable and can be carried by birds, blown around by the wind with dust or carried down streams and rivers, being left behind perhaps when floods recede, to start life in a new place.'

'If this coconut is so peaceful how come it's killing off my calves?' asked Charlie in pursuit of further enlightenment.

'Well,' I said 'maybe the animal swallows some of the spores when grazing and then gets a knock, especially over one of the big muscles on the hip or shoulder. The spore finds the bruised muscle to its liking, hatches out and starts multiplying at a fast rate; it now looks like a short bar instead of a coconut. Another theory is that the spores get in through a small scratch of some sort. Hard to say, but the result is clear enough.'

'Too right,' said Charlie. 'I don't suppose there's a lot a man can do about it — this creek comes from way back and your guess is as good as mine as to what happens up there.'

'Fortunately,' I said, 'there is a very efficient vaccine against the disease and if you have your calves treated, say around September, you should have nothing to fear, but it will have to be done each and every year as the spores can last for twenty years or more on the ground.'

Charlie seemed a bit disappointed when I told him I didn't have a supply of vaccine, because this was the first time I had diagnosed the disease. However, I said, 'I'll have some within a day or so even if it is Christmas and we'll treat the survivors.'

'If there are any to treat,' commented my neighbour.

Three days later I returned and administered the appropriate dose to the five remaining calves. They looked healthy enough although I warned that it could take around a week for immunity to build.

As I left the shed after washing up Charlie presented me with a jar of cream and a bunch of dahlias, apologising for disturbing our Christmas. A nice gesture I though and typical of that time.

I soon established a list of properties on which I encountered Blackleg and henceforth in September each year I carried out a protective innoculation programme. This was highly successful but the infection kept spreading to other properties, chiefly I presumed, down waterways. It was an on-going situation.

Cricket, Cars and other Things

In my last year at school in Glasgow in 1939 I had achieved some distinction as a cricketer, but the war years had allowed only occasional chances to play. My evolution was thus placed on hold for a decade, which in the normal course of events could have been rewarding. However, I soon discovered many keen supporters of the game in the Bay of Islands and I determined if possible to make good some of the lost opportunities of my youth. Some of the local players, like myself, were ex-servicemen keen to participate again in a sport long denied them. The younger generation was also enthusiastic. Northland College, the local secondary school, contributed two teams to the district cricket league which included teams from Kerikeri (called the citrus boys), Kawakawa, Kaikohe, Okaihau and Ohaeawai. When I could I turned out for Ohaeawai.

It soon became evident that as I was one of the players who lived nearest to our field of play I became honorary groundsman, as well as opening bowler. Now cricket is played in spring and summer and during these seasons the grass on the rich volcanic soil could almost be seen growing. Quite a few hours each week were needed to keep the playing square in acceptable condition. The outfield was another matter, and the best that could be done was to persuade the farmer whose property adjoined the sports ground to graze a large flock of sheep there as often as he could manage. This did not happen as often as we would have liked, with the result that batsmen more often attempted 'sixes' than 'fours' as balls driven along the ground rapidly lost momentum beyond the mown square.

Another problem with sheep was the cricket pavilion, which in those days was fairly primitive — a corrugated iron shack with a dilapidated wooden floor. The doors of this so-called pavilion were insecure and the sheep soon found it an ideal place to shelter from the heat of summer. When so doing they also did other things and visiting players were loud in their complaints. The droppings of sheep and the whites of cricketers were not particularly compatible, to say nothing of the not unpleasant but rather irrelevant woolshed odour which pervaded the place.

Nonetheless, the ladies rallied round with morning and afternoon teas, often of a standard city players, better provided for in other ways, would have envied. We played cricket with vigour and enthusiasm. Success in the earlier years was limited, mainly through domination by the better-funded and equipped Kaikohe teams, who also had some very good players like much-feared fast bowler, Vic Pearson, and wicket-keeper Stew Munro.

It was customary each alternate New Year for an Ohaeawai team, often including a few 'ring-ins' from elsewhere, to travel to Ruawai on the eastern shore of the extensive Kaipara harbour. It was a journey made to do battle with a team sponsored and captained by 'Mac' McGregor, a friend and colleague who was in charge of veterinary affairs in that part of the world. The following year the gesture was reciprocated with a team from Ruawai travelling to Ohaeawai for yet another vigorously contested game. But cricket is also a convivial sport and with the matches being played at the gate of the year and captained by two Scots at that, it was not surprising that there was a fairly strong social input later in the day when the last ball had been bowled and the sun had started to sink in the west.

I well remember one post-match function at Ruawai when, as the evening wore on, tongues loosened and the convivial tempo increased. Finey Sigley, who with me opened the bowling for Ohaeawai, inquired of a local, 'What's the chance of getting a few toheroas now we're down here — they reckon there's plenty?'

'Too right,' was the response, 'but you have to know where to go and at this time of night you wouldn't get within a bull's roar of them and most likely you'd get bogged in the sand as well.'

'But there's a moon,' persisted Finey.

'And,' said our opening batsman, 'my old man's pretty high up in the fisheries game in Wellington, so if I give the local inspector a ring he might just put us on the right track and keep us out of the bog.'

There was much laughter. All this seemed a bit unlikely but, believe it or not, the local inspector must have had a guilty conscience or was half asleep. He agreed. He said he would meet us at Dargaville, which was on our way home and was where he lived. It was also fairly convenient to the beach where we hoped toheroas rested in large numbers.

After a few for the road, two carloads of cricketers bid farewell to our hosts, promising retribution next year. We set off homewards along the Ruawai flats, across the Northern Wairoa river bridge and into Dargaville. True to his promise, at the appointed rendezvous stood a tall man of sallow complexion wearing a tartan jacket and hat to match, for the mist rising off the river made things a bit chilly. He did not look all that pleased for, after all, it was now after half-past-ten.

'Follow me!' said our guide as he climbed into his truck and set off on a course parallel to the murky river. Our number one car complied, and the one I was in soon followed, although there was a bit of a delay when some cricket gear fell out of the back seat onto the road.

We rounded a few corners in convoy but, as I have said, there was a bit of mist coming off the river and things weren't all that clear. Our driver had had a pretty good innings both out in the middle and at the after-match social, and maybe he wasn't as perceptive as he otherwise might have been. Anyhow, we tailed the red light ahead expecting soon to hear the roar of surf. After a while I remarked that it seemed a long way. About the same time we passed a signpost saying that the Waipoua forest was only another 15 miles up the road. Also about the same time the red light ahead disappeared off to the right into a farm driveway, the driver of the vehicle to which the light was attached apparently having arrived home.

Sadly we returned to Dargaville hoping to make some sort of contact with our cricketing mates and perhaps beg, borrow or steal a few of the delectable shellfish which by then they had no doubt collected.

Dargaville was as silent as the proverbial tomb and if any of the locals were around they were keeping to themselves. Much chastened we began the long trip home. I later learned that the other car had returned with two sacks of toheroas. I am afraid that it was not a good day for the cricketers in the car I was in. We lost one nil at cricket and two nil at toheroas!

Things improved a lot in the world of cricket though, for by 1954 Ohaeawai became Bay of Islands champions, a victory to which I felt I, with the redoubtable Finey Sigley, made some contribution as a player as well as erstwhile groundsman.

It was always a bit of a problem to get away to play and it was not unusual for my wife to arrive bringing news of some ailing animal somewhere. At other times a farmer passing by and recognising me on the field of play fielding on the boundary, might stop to discuss a problem. I recall removing a fish hook from a pet rabbit's ear in the pavilion, which was hardly suitable as a cricket pavilion let alone a surgery. I was not alone in mixing business with pleasure. A local man of the cloth was a cricketer of enthusiasm and no mean ability. Occasionally a wedding or some other vital church function clashed with Saturday cricket, creating a clash of loyalties. A rapid change of habit from white to black, some reorganisation of the batting order, a blessing of the happy couple, reverse habit change, and perhaps a well-struck half-century flowed in rapid order, with still time for a visit to the reception when stumps had been drawn.

When the day's labours on the cricket field had been concluded it was customary for most of the participants to quench their thirst, celebrate their victory or drown their sorrows. The hotel at Kerikeri is one I recall with particular pleasure, perhaps because of its rural atmosphere, pleasant setting and the games with the local club. It sometimes happened that farmers turned cricketers — and there were more than a few — like Cinderella forgot the passage of time. They arrived home to find cows with tense udders expectantly awaiting the creak of a gate or bark of a dog telling them that afternoon milking was nigh. At such times, when the predicament of the team member became known and the bewitching hour of six was upon us, volunteers were not lacking. Cricketers turned cockies descended on the cowshed, no doubt to the confusion and perhaps alarm of the cows being milked. I was never a participant in such episodes because I usually had to return home where a problem only a vet could solve often awaited.

One of the biggest advances in the treatment of animal diseases in the fifties was the increasing range and availability of the so-called ethical drugs — drugs available to the public only through a professional, or on the prescription of somebody qualified. The sulphonamides were particularly successful in treating the common diarrhoeas or scours of calves and a number of pig complaints. Mastitis, most likely the most common disease in the country, responded admirably to the antibiotic, penicillin. This came in gel form and was dispensed in small collapsible tubes. The contents could easily be squeezed through the teat canal into any quarter of the affected udder.

At first, penicillin for veterinary use was available only on prescription through vets. Farmers, politicians and firms seeking further business argued that this made the outlet too restrictive and pressure built for wider marketing channels. The result was that the drug became available virtually on demand.

While I could see the reasoning behind all this, for some areas were still starved of a veterinary presence, some interesting results were to follow. Farmers hailed penicillin as a new elixir and many felt that mastitis was now on the way out. Efforts to control the disease, such as through better shed hygiene, were placed on hold while pencillin was king. Now nature has never been one to give up easily. As bacteria and their viral cousins make up most living things it is likely that a meeting was held somewhere. Obviously it was decided that brother streptococcus, who to that time had conducted the mastitis operation with conspicuous success — but which was now being threatened by penicillin — should stand aside and allow brother staphlococcus a go. Staphlococcus was also well versed in the mastitis game but still had a few tricks to learn. Although penicillin also caused him a few headaches he was a survivor and it was felt he would do a good job.

The result was that farmers soon found that penicillin was not performing as well as it had been in the mastitis stakes because streptococcus was no longer running. His place had been taken by staphlococcus, helped by a few other brothers like corynebacterium and pseudomonas. The pharmaceutical industry had, of course, accepted this challenge and newer antibiotics effective against the latest invaders were soon devised. They were regularly produced to meet further challenges which nature evolved. The battle was, and is, a see-saw affair. Some human and animal diseases are well-controlled, but others such as mastitis, continue to persist in increasingly complex forms. It is commonly accepted that antibiotics in medical and veterinary practice have been over-used, sometimes through patient or owner pressure demanding a short term solution without regard for longer-term consequences.

One story illustrates my point. I had examined a pet dog suffering from eczema, a common canine skin complaint. Afterwards I was washing up in the bathroom of the farm house when I noticed a tube of penicillin-streptomycin combination I sometimes dispensed for stubborn mastitis cases on the window sill above the hand basin. On my return to the kitchen I inquired of the farmer's wife what the veterinary medicine was doing in her bathroom.

'Oh,' she replied, 'Joe reckons that stuff's just great when he cuts himself shaving — he uses it all the time.'

The tube in question bore the legend 'For Animal Use Only' but maybe my client reckoned he was a two-legged animal and maybe he was right. However, if he happened sometime to become affected with pneumonia or some other catastrophic illness, and his physician was concerned that his response to antibiotic therapy was less than expected, I wondered if the reason would be suspected.

As the 1950's progressed our grounds and house, now resplendent in its new coat of paint, made further progress. I built a passable stone wall around the circular drive with stones laboriously collected by wheelbarrow from our paddock. It emulated a practice, although by no means the skill, of early settlers and soldiers who constructed magnificent stone walls with every stone dovetailing with its neighbour. Many of these monuments to industry still stand and are much in evidence round Maungatapere near Whangarei. 'Dry stane dykes', as they were called, were common enough in Scotland but I saw nothing there which could match the excellence of their New Zealand counterparts.

The lawns were laid and surrounded by a concrete edge — a skill which took me a long time and a bit of frustration to acquire. A cattle stop was built at the road entrance to keep our small flock at home without the chore of opening and shutting the gate every time I went out or came in, which was often. We had acquired the sheep to control the grassy acres. Another cattle stop was needed to keep the sheep out of the cultivated garden. Trees, of a type we thought would do well, were planted on the banks of the stream, each one needing to be fenced off. We had found that sheep had a taste for many things apart from grass. I established a small vegetable garden near the back door and its prolific produce was a welcome addition to our diet for many years.

The canopy of oaks enclosed our stream, which was now visible although still subject to attack by willow and other weeds which needed constant control. To cap things off a daughter was born, and this once again turned my attention to interior renovation. A bedroom had to be relined in softboard, painted pale pink and a wardrobe built from rimu plywood later stained to emphasise its grain. I thought it all looked pretty good but then things you do yourself often look that way!

It was fast becoming apparent that my car was going to need early replacement. It was now 12 years old and suffering from its splayed front axle, using nearly as much oil as petrol, and having developed a disturbing habit with its electrics. Worn wiring resulted in all the lights being suddenly extinguished when they were needed most. For some time I had been reading the literature about the Landrover, then the only new four-wheel-drive vehicle available in the country. I also had the chance of observing one in action when a sheep farmer, who farmed some very steep hill country at Waimatenui, south of Kaikohe, transported me to the back of his farm. A bull he owned required my attention but could not easily be driven nearer home. I was impressed with the performance of this vehicle and determined to own one if I could. I was fairly short of cash and the price of £600 was nearly a year's salary. In the end we managed to scrape enough together and placed an order for the vehicle which, I was told, was on the water and could be expected within a month. This was quite satisfactory for the vehicle I was using really was getting a bit on the risky side. My board agreed to hire or purchase (I've forgotten which) the Secretary's Model A Ford to carry me over the few weeks until the Landrover arrived. This was the car in which John Phillips had met me when I first arrived and although I was not over-impressed with the prospect it appeared a better risk than the dangerous machine I was then using.

Things did not turn out quite as planned. The wharfies felt they deserved a better deal and Syd Holland, among others, thought they didn't. The ports closed up and my Landrover in Auckland Harbour may as well have been in Timbuctoo. This left me with the Model A in which in the end I travelled some 10,000 miles in the four months or so I was its driver.

Now this was a car with a personality. Unlike the V8, which could seldom be taken off a paved way because its high gearing caused its rear wheels to fail to grip on any slippery or unstable surface, the Model A could proceed across quite muddy places with impunity. Although a lot slower on the road, it was in some ways a step in the right direction.

However it did have a few disturbing habits. When stopped after a journey of any length it was inclined after half-a-minute or so, to shatter the silence with exploding gases somewhere within its vital parts. It so happened that at this time the chairman of my Board, Hubert Hatrick, had been pressing me to submit a monthly report summarising my activities during the period under review. I had resisted this bureaucratic type of exercise for which I could see no justification. One day when I arrived to administer to his pigs, Hubert happened to be near the road gate which he opened to permit my entrance. I drove the short distance to the cowshed and disembarked while my chairman made his way up the drive to join me. At that point the car, as was sometimes its custom, produced an explosion which must have left Hubert with the feeling he was back in Gallipoli.

'That should cover this month's report,' I remarked as Hubert joined me. The subject was never raised again.

On another occasion my brother-in-law had been visiting us and I invited him to accompany me on a call I had to make to the other side of Kawakawa. He readily agreed and we completed the trip and its purpose without incident. On the return journey, as we bowled along the Moerewa flat at a good clip, there was a sudden crash. The car lost its equilibrium, developing a crab-like motion before coming to rest with a list like some damaged vessel at sea. For some reason one rear wheel had become detached, and driven by its own impetus had travelled up the wide entrance to the Moerewa freezing works for quite some distance. Maybe the wheel felt that the rest of the car should have followed it — I don't know. We retrieved the dissenting disc, jacked up the car and, after borrowing a couple of nuts from the wheel's neighbour, reconnected the missing wheel and proceeded on our way with much hilarity. A lesser car might have suffered some damage, but the Model A seemed to take such minor transgressions in its stride.

One day when work was done we decided that some shopping was necessary. Leaving our daughter in the capable hands of Mrs Mason across the road, we set off for Kaikohe, our nearest town and shopping centre some six miles away. The petrol tank in the Model A was located behind the dash and, unknown to me, had developed a small, almost microscopic leak. When the car was in motion this caused a miniscule bead of petrol to escape and proceed by gravity down the steering column. Normally this would have had little impact other than an economic one, but on the night in question the engine, which always ran fairly hot, decided to surpass itself. After about one third of our return journey had been completed I noticed a rise in temperature and a dull glow beginning to shine at the foot of the steering column where it disappeared through the floor. Nor was this all. The occasional globule of petrol proceeded on its way down the steering column and on making contact with the hot metal exploded with a white flash resembling a small firework. We found this display of pyrotechnics rather disturbing and while on a number of occasions I had faced an early demise while in pursuit of my calling, the idea of being incinerated in a Model A Ford had little appeal. We abandoned the car and became hitchhikers, reaching home a little later than expected, but at least we got there!

Next day I had the erring vehicle recovered. My mechanic remarked that they always ran hot — something to do with the timing he thought. He fiddled around a bit inside the bonnet and pronounced the car as good as new, although he did feel I should do something about the leaky petrol tank. I agreed wholeheartedly, but a couple of days later the wharf strike ended and within the week my new Landrover, resplendent in its canvas cover and gray paint covering rust-proof panels, was proudly parked outside our house. I drove three Landrovers covering some 280,000 miles, and for me they never put a wheel wrong. My transport problems, possibly my greatest obstacle of the early years, had at last been solved. The Landrover, however, was not the ideal personal vehicle because its short wheel base and positive springing gave a bumpy ride. The canvas canopy was by no means airtight and the draughts and winds of winter sometimes made things unpleasant. However, it had its compensations — children could be put to bed in the tray and quite long distances covered before they woke.

The great asset was the four-wheel-drive which allowed me to go places I had not gone before. My farmer clients were greatly interested in my new acquisition because it was one of the first to appear in the district. I suspect that they sometimes combined business with pleasure. If my patient happened to be out the back somewhere, my client would climb expectantly into the passenger seat. In the past a tractor or even a saddled horse would have been provided for my transport.

An annual duty which soon became my lot was that of officiating at local sporting events in a professional capacity. What had happened in this respect in the hundred-odd years before my arrival I never knew.

One such function was the Kaikohe race meeting which, although not attracting the best gallopers in the country, the ones that did come and their supporters made up in enthusiasm what they lacked in ability. They managed to traverse the circular track on a paddock owned by local farmer, Jack Byers, showing a good turn of speed. I had known Jack for some time, not only as a client but also as a member of the Northland College Board of Governors. Jack had another skill, which I am sure if he had developed it would have taken him far. Perched high on a platform built in a fork of a large macrocarpa tree he gave a professional commentary on the progress of the equines competing in every race on the card. With his voice amplified by the loudspeaker system I don't think that I have heard a better performance in this exacting calling. The big event of the day was the Kaikohe Cup, the impressive trophy being presented by Mayor Guy with due ceremony and acclamation.

I do not recall my professional services ever being needed at the races but the same could not be said of the Waimate Show, held annually in November in the most attractive showgrounds just over the hill from Ohaeawai. If the puriris which studded the paddocks had been oaks this place could have been part of rural England, a conclusion reached by many early settlers and missionaries including Charles Darwin who spent Christmas at Waimate in 1835. The oldest oak tree in New Zealand, planted in 1824 and transferred from Paihia to its present site in 1831, is nearby. Also there is the historic church of St John the Baptist, originally built by the lay missionaries in 1831, and since maintained in pristine condition by their descendants and now the Historic Places Trust. Nearby is the old vicarage built for missionary and gunsmith George Clarke in 1832, and now maintained by the same National Trust. Much more has been written about the early history of Ohaeawai and Waimate North by authorities far better informed than myself. I sometimes attended weddings, funerals and other functions at Waimate North and indeed do to this day. For me it has always been a pleasure to work, worship and play in a place so beautiful where the ghosts of the past never seem too far away.

But to return to the show! Show day was no doubt an event of the year, a meeting place for young and old and catering for a wide range of tastes and preferences. The programme was perhaps dominated by the equestrian events, whose competitive schedule kept riders and judges busy from early morning to quite late in the evening. In a professional sense, it was the jumping events which caused me the greatest concern. International rules seemed to apply in some ways but they most certainly did not in others. My chief cricitism was that most of the hurdles were built in such a way as would have done credit to the palisades and other fortifications built around the nearby heavily defended pas over a century before.

Large logs bound together with fencing wire had no give. Although not very high, woe and betide any horse unwise or unskilled enough to fail to clear such an obstacle. With forefeet suddenly checked, the horse usually crashed to ground nose first, propelling the rider over its head into the relative safety of the open spaces ahead. Sometimes though, the unfortunate horse completed a full somersault and then the rider was not so lucky. The full weight of the steed descended upon him or her with serious consequences. In most cases, it was the horse which suffered, for on landing the neck often twisted to one side, leading to a fracture of the vertebral column and instant death. I saw a number of these accidents early on. Later, partly at my instigation, commonsense prevailed and hurdles which collapsed on impact were provided, significantly reducing the risk to horse and rider. It also improved the sport, for now higher obstacles of greater variety could be provided, stimulating greater competitiveness and spectator interest.

With so many equines assembled, some having come a long way over indifferent roads and suffering changes in their dietary routine, it was inevitable that digestive disturbances would surface. I had to treat quite a few colic cases. There were also some cuts and bruises associated with the loading and unloading routine and these too needed the vet. It was not unusual while our family was viewing the selection of exquisite blooms on display in the hall, for the tranquil hour to be interrupted by the blare of a loudspeaker requesting the vet's urgent presence.

I do not mean to give the impression that these shows were a series of veterinary catastrophes. Indeed, only a few animals needed the vet and the complaints were often minor. However, many of the competitors were children who showed great concern when injury or illness befell their much-loved charges. I often had to comfort those whose temporarily incapacitated competitor was forced out of the running, making the trip, for that day at least, unavailing.

In the 1950's farming in New Zealand was becoming more rewarding. This was partly due to the efforts of willing ex-servicemen who had been established on their farms by a grateful government. They were now eager to prove themselves, supported by an older generation which was set in its ways from their their methods having stood the test of time. The idea of a sheep farm in Hawkes Bay was paradise to many.

In such a setting, the demand for veterinary service of an ever-increasing livestock population was strong. For the greater part of the decade there was a chronic shortage of professional staff. The busy season was a particularly trying time and it was the custom for veterinary students undergoing training in Australia to return during their holiday break, ostensibly to gain training in the field, but more accurately to fill gaps in the existing veterinary establishment struggling to cope. I was always a bit uneasy about pitching these students in at the deep end. By carefully monitoring the calls and clients they attended, and by a degree of consultation before they left, they served a useful purpose. They also had to show an initiative and skill in public relations which I had never been allowed to practice in my student days. My students, most of whom were ex-servicemen, were still young, and the exuberance of youth overcame many of the physical and technical difficulties involved. I do not recall many complaints from clients, so the system seemed to work.

Some of my students must have been impressed by their lot for on graduation one or two joined our veterinary staff. One was Alan Twaddle, who filled a vacancy we had established at Kaeo. Alan successfully managed the Kaeo branch for a number of years before transferring to the Bay of Plenty and higher things. With Whangaroa now having a vet, Hokianga felt a bit left out in the cold. However, we managed to secure the services of an Irish graduate appropriately called Billy O'Brien. He was provided with a house at Rawene with a magnificent outlook over the Hokianga Harbour towards the setting sun. Although the work-load was not all that heavy, Billy found the roads and the isolation more than his family could bear and after a month or two they departed for more benevolent parts, and finally back to County Cork.

Billy O'Brien was eventually replaced by Ken Peters, an Englishman who, like myself, had been an officer in the Royal Army Veterinary Corps during the war. Ken emigrated to New Zealand in response to an advertisement we had placed in the *British Veterinary Record* but also had family connections with a well-known doctor in Kerikeri. Ken was established at Kaikohe where he operated with the help of a number of assistants recruited as available. The Kaikohe branch handled the Hokianga, Kaikohe and Okaihau areas and with Kerikeri previously surrendered to Alan Twaddle, my workload was considerably reduced, on paper anyway. Increasing demand and preventitive programmes like brucellosis inoculation, and later bovine tuberculosis, filled the illusory gap created.

On a Wednesday night in summer and fall, when the fish were running right, Ken Peters and I headed out to sea. Around seven o'clock we joined a band of keen anglers and also rank amateur fishermen on board the *Owaka* at Paihia wharf. Under the skilled hand of Edmund Lane, a one-time coastal dairy farmer and client, our vessel used to move across the usually placid bay towards the places he thought the fish would be. They were at that, and it was a poor night which didn't yield half a sackful for us. Fish gutted, we returned inland across the deserted countryside and I crept gently to bed fearful that I might disturb my slumbering family.

Late Fifties

Let me begin this part with a story. Among other things I had brought back from Scotland was a Tam o' Shanter resplendent in its McGregor tartan, a clan of which the name Stirling is a sect. It had not been my practice to wear

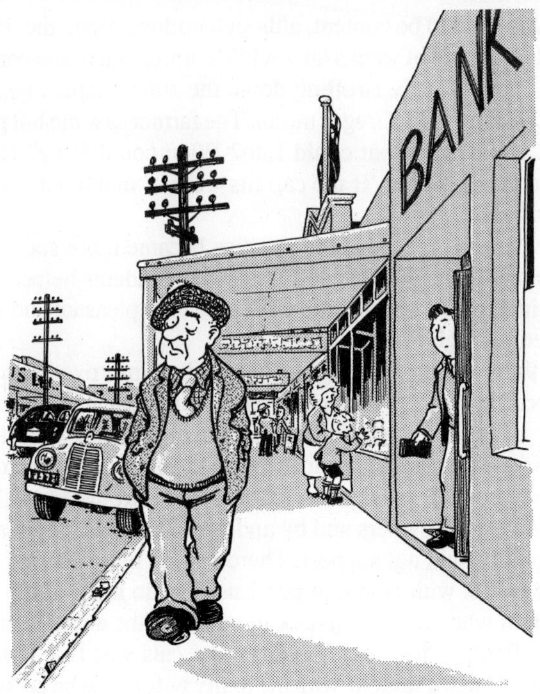

a hat of any sort in New Zealand, in the belief that it might encourage premature baldness. This was a failing to which the male members of the family tree was subject, but of which I had so far shown no sign. However, one cold and frosty morning before the sun was up I had a call to an ailing cow. I donned my new Scottish hat, which I must say proved comfortable and a welcome protection from the early morning chill.

Anxious to preserve the pristine condition of my headgear I removed it while I attended the cow. When I finished I must have been distracted because I forgot to reclaim my cap. I returned home in the brilliant sunshine which often follows a frosty morning, and was about to leave again after a sustaining breakfast when the lady of the house, pointing to an empty hook in the hall inquired,

'Where is your new tartan bonnet?'

Where indeed? I was only too well aware where the hat was and that evening rang the farmer concerned to inquire if he had recovered it from the bench beside the milk vat in his cowshed.

'Can't say I saw it,' said my client, 'but I'll have another look in the morning — don't think it's there though. Tell you what … if I find it I'll drop it in. How's that?'

With this I had to be content, although nothing along the lines suggested transpired. A couple of weeks later while coming out of the bank in Kaikohe I saw my client bravely strolling down the street resplendent in a Tam o' Shanter styled in the McGregor tartan. The farmer saw me but passed, stony-faced and unmoved. What could I do? What could I say? He had clearly interpreted the metaphor 'If the cap fits wear it' in a much more literal and practical sense.

As the decade proceeded the practice became more stabilised although still occasionally plagued by staff shortages. Students helped to fill the gap left from time to time and a number of these very pleasant and willing young men passed through my hands.

I also think my professional technique had improved, largely no doubt because practice makes perfect or something near to it. I was anxious to develop a service to the pets of the district, although it was a field in which my experience was limited, and I received little encouragement from my board. They considered the service had been brought into being for the benefit of livestock owners and by and large it should stay that way. It was a philosophy I could not support. There was no other service available to a distraught owner with an ailing pet. I used to do most of my small animal work at night when it was too dark to attend to the animals of the fields.

One difficulty I had with the dogs and cats was that I was usually by myself unless I had a student with me or my wife could be persuaded to help. Pet owners were unsatisfactory nurses as the sight of the blood or internal organs of a family member often led to a white-faced erstwhile assistant making a hasty exit or as occasionally happened, collapsing on the floor of the surgery. The choice was to continue ministrations to the anaesthetised patient or transfer them to the unconscious owner.

It was not only pets that ended up on the operating table. I recall that one night after dinner a well-known local sheep farmer, Marsden by name, rang to say that he had a stud Southdown ewe which he was not able to lamb. Sheep farmers, unlike their dairy farm colleagues, were mostly well versed in correcting any of the usual deviations preventing an ovine birth. By the time they came to my attention, which wasn't often, I could usually expect that the impediment to birth was difficult. The case in point was just that, for the pelvis of the two-tooth Southdown was far too small to permit the passage of the unborn lamb. I could barely get three fingers beyond the bony pelvis to assist the birth, far less a hand.

Because of the better lighting and water supply I had suggested to my client that it might be wise to bring the patient to the surgery, but when the woolly ewe was placed on the small operating table I doubted the wisdom of my advice. A Caesarian operation was the only hope of success and we decided to go ahead.

The first step was to remove the matt of tangled down fleece in which many thistles and other things were trapped. Using hand shears and working in shifts we finally managed to expose the white and pink skin.

Once this preparation was completed, the paravertebral anaesthetic in place, and the proposed line of incision defined by a streak of crystal violet dye, it did not take too long to proceed with the operation and deliver a large, struggling and snuffling ram lamb with the brown face characteristic of his breed. For safety, and because there was nowhere else to put him, I placed the new arrival in the sink. The stitching of uterus, muscles and skin took a lot longer though, but was nearly finished when Marsden drew my attention to the fact that the son in the sink was breathing irregularly. I abandoned mother and turned my attention to her offspring but, alas, too late. Despite frantic clearing of the air passages and artificial respiration, life could not be sustained. Perhaps if I had had better equipment or paid more attention to son rather than mother things might have been better. Being a one man band is never easy. I was down 1-0.

I finished the suturing and after administering an antibiotic injection as a shield against infection I helped my client carry the patient to his truck parked in the moonlit drive. The ewe lived to breed again so I guess the game ended one-all. Could have been better, could have been worse ... but such is life.

With our daughter now at school I was about to be introduced to the New Zealand education system.

The Ohaeawai School, pleasantly situated near the village church, and only a short distance from the historic rock of Taiamai, had a grassy paddock for play, unlike the hard bitumen of the playground I attended as a boy and which often removed skin and more from the knees of sprawling schoolboys. A swimming pool was soon to provide an added amenity, although the nearby creek had pools of varying depths suitable for beginners and experts alike.

It was not long before I was elected a member of the school committee. I had imagined that the school committee might have had some input into the syllabus and the way knowledge was instilled into youthful heads. However, I soon discovered that the committee was a semi-social organisation, often more concerned with the raising of funds for a new piece of equipment not provided by a benevolent government. It was more concerned with providing transport for some outing or other, rather than discussing more basic things like reading, spelling, arithmetic or homework. If a teacher robbed a bank or did something worse the committee could voice disapproval. In my view, too little emphasis was placed on core subjects and too much on marginal or peripheral activities. School, I think, was never meant to be fun for which long holidays are allowed. I believe poor attainment levels in basic subjects, along with poor discipline which often encouraged children to argue instead of conform, is the root cause of a number of this country's social problems.

On the school role was a significant number of Maori students. I must say that in a district where Maoris abounded and still had strong historical links with the many conflicts of not so long ago, racism did not exist. But officialdom seemed to regard the Maori as different, needing to be taught in a different way with concessions bestowed upon them. Too often the Maori was being gently persuaded along lines for which they showed an aptitude, such as their own language, arts, crafts and music. All of these provided cultural outlet for inherent talent but provided no preparation for the often mundane world of western materialism from which New Zealanders of any colour find it difficult to divorce themselves. It was, and is in my view, a disservice to all things Maori. The soft approach, along with misplaced cultural and racial emphasis and an attitude of concession, is in fact a denial of the equality that all races, not least of all the Maori, appear to seek.

You may well question my qualifications to pronounce on these things. I've played sport with Maoris, I have worked for Maoris as my clients, and Maoris have worked for me on my land. I have supervised the work of Maoris and debated issues of the day with them. My children attended a school whose pupils were about half Maori. I found little difference in intellect, and still less in a sense of human values. There was certainly nothing requiring special treatment or concession which was, in my experience, never asked or called for by the members of this talented race.

The Problem of Hydatid Disease

As the the decade drifted on my interests turned to a variety of things. One campaign in which I was to become involved in increasing measure was the one to control hydatid disease in animals and people.

I had always felt that the vet should exploit his training to a maximum and, where possible, become particularly involved in the aspects of his calling which had a direct link with human health and well-being. The inelegant term 'zoo noses' is given to collectively describe that group of animal diseases which can be transmitted to people. There are around 30 such diseases in New Zealand, including brucellosis and hydatids.

Hydatid disease normally pursues a cycle starting with a small flat tapeworm about a quarter-inch long found attached to the small intestine of the dog or fox where it takes about seven weeks to grow up. The last segment of this small parasite becomes chock-full of about 500 eggs when it reaches maturity. This envelope of eggs finally detaches itself and passes out with the droppings of the dog onto the grass or garden or wherever. The envelope dries up and releases its bounteous contents to be spread by wind or water to other places. Along comes an ovine, bovine, porcine or caprine and picks up some eggs with the grass it fancies. The egg shell soon dissolves and the active little worms, or embryos as they are called, are like homing pigeons. Via the bloodstream they reach the liver, lungs, heart, brain or some other important place. Here they hook their little heads on to a spot they like and grow into a cyst which after a month or two looks like a thin-skinned table tennis ball. These cysts form other cysts inside themselves and these contain batteries of scolices or, if you like, heads of new tapeworms. If a dog eats infected offal, the little worms are keen to attach themselves to the canine intestine and start the programme all over again, completing the life cycle.

Humans can take the place of the sheep in the cycle. People handle dogs and dogs' coats are sometimes contaminated by their own droppings or those of their peers. Garden produce contaminated by an infected dog can cause grievous harm to its consumer if eaten raw and unwashed.

Sheep and other animals harbouring hydatid cysts appear to be able to carry large numbers without undue concern. I have seen livers looking more like a box of ping pong balls than a vital organ, but the animal seemingly healthy. People were generally not so lucky. The cyst or cysts cause chronic illness and extensive and sometimes repeated surgery is needed to effect a cure. From 1950 to 1953 some 58 people died from hydatid disease and 377 needed to be admitted to hospital for treatment. Here, to my thinking, was a challenge and an opportunity.

The situation in New Zealand was about the worst in the world. Only Iceland and some South American countries were worse. The reason was not hard to find. It had long been the custom that when sheep were killed for domestic use the liver and lungs were tossed to the dogs or left unprotected where any marauding canine could easily find a sustaining meal. It was clear to me that a two-pronged approach was needed. Firstly, dogs had to be denied access to infected and uncooked offal. Secondly, the tenacious parasites had to be removed from the intestines of dogs harbouring them. This was easier said than done. Arecoline tablets, which expelled the offending tapeworms, had long been distributed with new dog collars by itinerant rangers employed by local county councils when they called on farmers to register the dogs. But all dogs were not registered and the arecoline tablets had a rather violent purging action. Because of this the owners did not use the tablets. Large jars containing a number of years supply rested on ledges in woolsheds and other farm buildings. The habit of feeding raw offal to dogs was well ingrained, and dogs were often left to scavenge at will.

I came to the conclusion that if progress was to be made someone with authority — far greater than the part time rangers — would need to be employed to carry out dosing and at the same time instruct dog owners about safe feeding methods. County councils were the logical framework on which to build a hydatid control system. This, of course, was original thinking as no local body had ever before directly taken any part in measures to control animal disease. The thinking had always been that such measures were the responsibility of central government.

Someone had to start so I convened a meeting of all organisations I thought might be interested and helpful, including the County Council, Federated Farmers, Women's Division of the same organisation, dairy companies, Department of Agriculture and a few others. I was fortunate that the chairman of the Bay of Islands County Council at that time was Charles Frederick Jones. Charlie farmed quite a large, immaculately presented sheep farm of some 500 acres at Pakaraka, dominated by a gracious two-storeyed home called *Ngaheia*. It had 10 rooms and had been built more than 100 years before for Joseph Marsden Williams, the eleventh and youngest son of Reverend Henry Williams, the pioneer missionary. Charlie, being a sheep farmer and a perceptive one at that, was aware of the seriousness of the problem and threw his weight behind the idea. Without this support I do not think progress would have been made. A steering committee was formed with myself as chairman, and after a lot of discussion it was decided that a full-time hydatids control officer would be appointed as an employee of the County Council.

This was a momentous decision, for although some other schemes were already in operation I think it fair to say that the Bay of Islands scheme became the prototype for the whole country.

The position of hydatid control officer was filled by Blundell Wynyard in late 1958. Blundell was a conscientious man with a background of farming who had a love of dogs and a lot of experience handling them.

The modus operandi decided was that all dogs would be periodically dosed with arecoline to induce purging and hopefully expel the tapeworms. The faecal samples were recovered and examined microscopically. Dogs were therefore, theoretically at least, cleared of their parasitic burden and identified if infected. Preventive measures, such as modifying the feeding system, could then be applied to those infected.

A microscope was funded by the dairy company and roadside dosing strips constructed. Council graders removed the surface growth, leaving bare soil from which matter expelled from the dogs could be collected and placed in plastic containers for further examination. Blundell's wife became the technician operating from their Paihia home and soon acquired the skill needed to identify the parasites. The scheme was a good example of local ingenuity and cooperation.

About the same time the seriousness of the hydatids situation began to attract the attention of the government and it was decided to form a National Hydatids Council to coordinate local effort, operated through local bodies. The stated objective was to guard human health in New Zealand and assist the economy by reducing the rejection rate of infected offal.

When the personnel of the proposed council were announced I noted with concern that no independent veterinary representative was included. I felt this was a serious omission as the problem was primarily a veterinary one and should have had appropriate professional veterinary input. The original Bill was referred to a committee of the House of Representatives for comment and I drew the attention of the New Zealand Veterinary Association to the prevailing situation. As a result, I was asked to make submissions on this point. The submission must have been successful for when the structure of the inaugural National Hydatids Council was announced room was made for a representative of the Veterinary Association. Although I did not especially seek it, I was asked to fill this vacancy. Because my absences from the practice could cause a few problems I was hesitant to accept. However, my colleagues and my board also felt I should contribute so I finally accepted and a new field of experience and endeavour opened for me.

The work entailed a meeting in Wellington about once a month, meaning a two-day absence. The flights to and from the north were not always smooth and I recall on several occasions the Dakota passing through the saddles in the hills south of Kaikohe and viewing the bush-clad summits from below rather than the more usual bird's eye panorama from above. I was often relieved to descend to a waiting wife at the airport ready to take me home. Sometimes the mists were even thicker and then the course was up the western coastline. Flying low over that rugged place I used to marvel at the wild breakers from the Tasman expending themselves at last on beach or rocky shore.

There was also a lighter side. I remember being tapped on the shoulder by an elderly lady seated behind me during a flight to Whangarei.

'I think the back door is open,' she informed me. 'Perhaps you should tell the pilot?'

This seemed a good idea for there was indeed no-one else to tell. Looking back I saw the door swinging disconcertingly on its hinges, looking as if was about to part company with the aircraft.

The pilot did not seem unduly upset and told me to lean over and give it a good bang. This had the desired effect and the pilot rewarded myself and the lady with an extra barley sugar from a bag he kept in his hip pocket. These were usually used to help alleviate the discomfort in passengers' ears resulting from changes in pressure when the aircraft descended.

Not all local bodies were enthusiastic about hydatid control. Control officers had to be appointed and trained and people found to do the training. A central testing station was established at Taieri, where vacant accommodation was available, and this handled all the faecal samples nationwide, reporting results back to individual authorities for follow-up action.

In the midst of all the progress, I identified a few cases where self-interest was clearly placed above the common good. At one of the first meetings of the National Hydatids Council I attended I moved a resolution to the effect that the campaign would sustain significant impetus if farmers could be credited with the proceeds from the offal of stock they sent for slaughter. The freezing companies had never paid for such offal, claiming that such a move would mean an upward move in killing charges. It was a premise which I thought was as unrealistic as unethical. The purpose of my resolution was that if a farmer had a high incidence of hydatid infestation in his stock it would naturally be reflected in a penalty caused through rejection of infested liver and lungs, especially the former. The farmer would therefore be encouraged to improve disease control. Surprisingly, the resolution was lost when put to the vote. Some farmer members were also members of freezing company directorates and maybe they were afraid of rocking the boat. Who can tell? Things are not always as straightforward as they seem. Despite a few invitations, freezing companies declined membership of the Council, notwithstanding the fact that in cash terms they would be the chief beneficiaries of success in the campaign which was now under way. It was an attitude as introvertive as it was naive.

The first chairman of the Council was Ira Cunningham, a distinguished veterinarian who was Assistant Director General of Agriculture. He later became the first Dean of the newly established veterinary faculty at Massey University. The first executive officer was Alan Laing, a veterinarian of long service within the Department of Agriculture.

I also soon became associated with the research side of the campaign which was of the highest importance. This was a unique experience which led me into another world.

The director of the Hydatid Research Unit was a bespectacled vet called Michael Gemmell who was employed by the powerful and wide-ranging Medical Research Council. The Council had for some reason become the academic force behind the campaign and accepted the responsibility for the running of a research unit which had a useful link with the testing station and was located quite close to it.

The Hydatid Research Council, on which I represented the National Hydatids Council, met infrequently and did not have a lot to do with influencing policy. Sir Charles Hercus, the Chairman, was sometimes receptive but like most true academics he was happy enough if his unit churned out its quota of well-presented technical literature, even if it did not always include practical information relating to how the tapeworm parasites could be controlled and eradicated. I was always impatient with the fact that results were not quickly achieved. In the end, progress was indeed made in many aspects but the route was perhaps more tortuous and ponderous than it needed to have been.

However, I made many friends in Dunedin and their hospitality at least could not be faulted. I recall attending a meeting in the depths of winter when my flight was diverted to Invercargill because of fog and frost and snow. It was late at night when I finally arrived in Dunedin by bus, cold and tired and hungry. I was met by Michael Gemmell who had arranged a place for me at his club, also regularly inhabited by many distinguished academics from that Edinburgh of the south, as Dunedin was sometimes called. In my bedroom was a Victorian sideboard of mahogany on which rested a covered tray of sandwiches, a decanter of malt Scotch, a crystal glass, a vacuum flask of coffee and a small silver jug of cream. For decoration a single red rose reposed in a silver vase. In the four-poster bed between the stiff, starched sheets I discovered a hot water bottle of stoneware. Old world hospitality indeed!

On another occasion we had enjoyed an agreeable dinner featuring a steak for which the hotel in which we were staying was renowned. Afterwards I remarked that if Dunedin was as Scottish as it claimed to be, then haggis should have been on the menu. My remark was overheard by the waiter serving coffee and he, no doubt anxious to promote his city's versatility, assured me that the cook downstairs was as expert as any in the homeland in manufacturing the Scottish delicacy. The waiter added that if I really wanted to pursue the haggis question I should visit the cook, an expatriate Scot from Aberfeldy. This cheerful chef, after reviewing the latest advances made by the Scottish National Party, told me that as a token of our meeting he would prepare a haggis and send it to me by air.

About a week later the National Airways depot in Kaikohe advised that a parcel had arrived from Dunedin. The contents appeared to have leaked, for a mixture of grease and other things had permeated the enclosing paper wrapping and had also involved several other packages travelling in the same aircraft. The none-too-happy airways agent requested the rapid uplifting of the offending package.

Why all this should have happened I do not know. Perhaps changes in air pressure had been too much for the haggis. We did in fact eat most of the ruptured haggis with plenty of turnip and mashed potato and found it quite delectable.

An important function of the National Hydatids Council was good public relations for the success of the campaign importantly depended upon the continuing support of dog-owning farmers and city dog owners. Dogs owned by the latter were a special danger. They could become infected during holiday time in the country and they often had close human contact, especially with children.

Council meetings were held far and wide, from Warkworth in the north to Invercargill in the south. This gave me the chance to visit places to which I might not otherwise have gone, and to meet many interesting and dedicated people. In Wellington I met a number of Ministers of Agriculture and even shook the hand of Walter Nash. One daunting assignment I had was to address the annual conference of the Women's Division of Federated Farmers at New Plymouth; they had agreed to sponsor and promote the campaign for a year. If there were any men around I did not see them. When I had stopped speaking they must have been impressed for they all clapped and the president gave me a cookery book as a memento of the occasion.

The Council itself had a few characters of note, none more so than Les Cameron, a farmer from the Wairarapa who represented the Counties on Council and pursued the campaign, despite indifferent health, as if it was an operation of war. When he couldn't sleep, which was often, Les thought nothing of ringing his M.P. Keith Holyoake, in the middle of the night to bring some matter to his attention. Another time Les was confined to a wheel chair but this did not deter him from planning to attend a hydatids related meeting in Dunedin where he was regarded with awe and a good deal of apprehension. The air hostess, who had promised to ensure that the Dunedin-bound farmer was loaded complete with chair on his appropriate flight, forgot all about him. She left him parked on the airport concourse. When Les discovered that the flight had departed without him his ire was absolute. The airport manager and a number of lesser beings were summoned and left in no doubt of the angry farmer's opinion of the service provided by the national airline. Luckily, Les still managed to arrive in Dunedin on time.

It surprised me a bit to find so many farmers who appeared to spend the entire working week in the capital representing this or that. I formed the opinion that status, and the modicum of power which such functions bestowed, were more significant to some than the contribution their limited competence allowed them to make.

I was a member of the National Hydatids Council for over a decade, and there naturally were changes. Council had always been involved in the control of a large tapeworm called Taemia hydatigena. This tapeworm also inhabited the small intestine of dogs, with sheep the secondary host. The migrating parasites often caused damage and consequent rejection. Another emerging problem was Taemia ovis, another large tapeworm in dogs. When the cysts appeared in the muscles of sheep it could cause condemnation of the whole carcase, a serious monetary loss for the farmer. It became clear that offal or the carcase of the sheep could not safely be fed to dogs unless it had been thoroughly cooked, or deep frozen for at least a week.

From 1946 to 1949, 57 people died through hydatid disease and many more suffered the anguish of surgery and hospitalisation, by 1986 to 1989 the death rate had fallen to only two. I left the Council in 1972 with a letter of thanks from the Minister of Agriculture but, far more important, with the knowledge that I had played a part in saving the lives of some and misery to many more. It was a stimulating and productive experience.

More Adventures and Challenges

Meantime, trips away or no, my practice still needed my constant attention, bringing me face to face with all sorts of off-beat veterinary adventures. On one occasion I was called out to see a lame bull on a farm at the end of a road winding its tortuous course into the hills in the back country beyond Kawakawa.

As I turned off the so-called main road at Taumarere, I could see black clouds with almost a straight baseline gathering in the west. There was lightning and no doubt thunder, although I could not hear it above my Landrover's engine and the crash of wheels on the pot-holed metalled road. Four miles later as I turned inland a few heavy splatters of rain on the windscreen were the precursor of more to come.

Five miles up the winding track into the hills beyond I drew up outside my client's white weatherboard house. A car was parked outside the house, and in the passenger seat sat a lady I took to be my client's wife. The farmer, who was about to enter the driver's seat, was dressed in a tight navy blue suit, white shirt and a red striped tie, not the sort of attire usually worn by farmers on the job, least of all in the back country behind Kawakawa.

'We're just off to Whangarei for the day,' my well-dressed client told me. 'I didn't know when you'd get here but the bull's tied up in the front garden,' he continued, indicating a two-year old Jersey bull with quite large horns. An attached rope passed through a ring in his nose and then around a post which was part of the garden fence.

I was not quite sure how it had been assumed that I could diagnose the lameness and possibly carry out some treatment without assistance, but the expectations of some of my clients were fairly high. However, on this occasion I had arrived before the bird had flown and although I could already see that the bull was lame in his left hind foot I informed his owner that I would need to make a closer examination before prescribing any treatment.

'No sweat there,' said my client. To my astonishment he vaulted the garden fence, grabbed the bull by the neck and the ring in his nose, and with a twist and a jerk which would have done credit to a wrestler he threw the patient to the ground. No doubt as surprised as I was, the bull submissively lay with his owner now draped over his neck. The cause of the lameness was not too hard to find, for embedded in the horny sole I detected a very bent and very rusty fence staple which I removed with a pair of strong forceps. An antibiotic injection discouraged further infection. My client moved off the patient's neck, dusted down his suit and encouraged his bull to move from garden to paddock, no doubt grateful to escape the attentions of his owner. He then climbed into the car beside his vaguely disapproving but not surprised wife telling me they'd better be off because if it rained a lot the road sometimes was flooded; quite large drops were beginning to fall.

'Grab yourself a cabbage from the vege garden round the back,' my client added as an afterthought, and in a shower of metal he departed for the city.

Twenty minutes later, having packed my gear in the car and picked a cabbage, I drove off. Sweeping round a corner back on level ground, I saw a sheet of water across my path. But not to worry! My Landrover with its four-wheel-drive was made for this sort of thing. It was quite exciting ploughing through water hazards with bow wave awash, like some ship at sea. But not this time. The flood was deeper than I thought and was soon up to floor level. The engine kept running, but my vehicle was now 30 degrees off course and still yawing; an impression of buoyancy was beginning to assert itself.

Looking to my right I could see a cascade pouring off the edge of the road and pouring into what had been a paddock, but was now a turbulent brown lake. The Bay of Islands wasn't all that far away and I felt I might soon be there — but no holiday trip this time! Luckily the angle of deviation to the right was not as great as it might have been and the off-front wheel made contact with a tree root and some manuka scrub, flattened by the torrent. It was enough to give the four-wheel-drive some purchase and take it into more shallow and peaceful waters before crawling ashore. With pumping heart I proceeded on my way, wondering if my client and his good lady were now at some destination they had not planned to be.

Another important veterinary condition which was specifically identified during this period was leptospirosis or 'redwater', caused by a bacterium of spiral form capable of causing severe illness in man as well as animals. My main association with this disease had been in calves which suddenly died around six weeks of age. The name 'redwater' was certainly an accurate description. On opening the abdominal cavity of a dead calf, the bladder was distended with blood-stained urine. By carrying out dozens of post mortems I was dicing with death. The tissues of afflicted calves were swarming with virulent bacteria, all too eager to change hosts through any abrasion.

In early days I used to prescribe ordinary salt in the milk or water as a preventative for surviving calves and this appeared of benefit. Perhaps it was only a perceived placebo and the incidence was going to drop anyway as immunity developed in the surviving calves.

It was soon discovered that pigs often harboured the causal organisms without themselves showing any signs. They could act as a source of infection for young bovines, and pigs and calves were often in close association on the farm. Human attendants were in contact with both. It was also found that the ubiquitous bacteria might cause abortion in adult cattle who could also be symptomless carriers. The threat to people was greatest therefore to those who attended pigs and those who milked. If their cows were milked in a herringbone cowshed, with the milker standing in a central pit with the cows above, a splash to the eyes from infective urine, or perhaps the flick of a contaminated tail across the face and eyes, were quite common. It was because of this that it became fashionable to dock the tails of cows, and although this removed the tool of relief from the cow in its continuous battle with irritating flies, it was of undoubted benefit to those who milked them.

Leptospirosis is a severe illness in people like a long-lasting severe influenza. In some ways it is very similar to brucellosis or undulant fever. Positive diagnosis is through a fairly complicated blood testing procedure and it is clear to me that in early days, when the cause had not been identified and no specific treatment prescribed, many must have survived only after long and debilitating illness. Some most likely did not survive at all. The number of deaths may have been relatively high for, proportionally, there was a greater man-stock association then than now, when far more live in the cities than before. Leptospirosis is still with us but it is now much more easily treated and diagnostic techniques are better. Vaccines are also now available to protect stock and people.

Life though was not all about the problems of animals and their two-legged masters. I continued to pursue my interest in cricket wherever possible and when Len Hutton's team was scheduled to play a test in Auckland's Eden Park at the end of March 1955 I decided it was compulsory viewing. Once again we booked in at the Star Hotel.

A baby sitter was acquired with some difficulty and we were all set to go. The night before our scheduled departure a storm of hurricane force swept in from the tropics and administered a severe beating to the north. We were lucky to reach our destination, for the way south was strewn with fallen trees.

In Auckland we were joined by fellow vet 'Mac' McGregor from Ruawai and enjoyed a day and more at the cricket. The game itself did not last all that long and it was constantly threatened by the fringes of the storm which had devastated the north. We had the doubtful pleasure of seeing the New Zealand team contribute the lowest ever test score — a mere 26. The speed of Tyson and Statham, with the guile of Appleyard superimposed, was all too much.

On arrival home we found that the family and their erstwhile guardian had had a wild night. The storm we had experienced the night before had turned on its tracks and battered the north once more. Our house had a window blown out and a well-established ponga fern in the front lawn was uprooted and unceremoniously dumped in the flooded creek below.

The hurricane did enormous damage. In Kerikeri, rows of gum trees planted for shelter were uprooted, crashing down and destroying fruit trees and burying power and telephone lines in the tangle of fallen branches. It was several days before services were restored and many months before the debris removed.

Back in the north the 1957-58 cricket season at local level also provided a pleasant diversion and our Ohaeawai team won the Bay of Islands championship. The result was still in doubt to the last when Ohaeawai engaged the powerful Kaikohe Eleven at Ohaeawai for the final and deciding encounter. Kaikohe had a population of well over 3,000 and was able to draw on that resource of manpower for its team. In the country, the availability of important contributors was too often compromised by the demands of milking, hay-making, shearing and the like, most of such activities taking place during the cricket season. However, on the day, the bowling of the home team was the trump card and although Kaikohe naturally blamed the pitch, the victory was conclusive. Victor and vanquished celebrated the occasion and the winding up of the season in the hotel at 'The Corner' for quite some time.

I managed to take over 100 wickets for the first time and I also played a game or two for the Bay of Islands in the Dargaville Shield competition for teams representing the northern counties. In this, the competition was stronger and my performance considerably less memorable but it was still very enjoyable.

The End of the Decade

As the decade drew to its close I began to develop an interest in farming in a personal sense rather than as a spectator vet. I had always kept a few sheep because our house was set in two stony acres. The flock of about ten was soon to multiply five-fold. The four or five acres of the Ohaeawai sports field where I played cricket in summer, became available for grazing. In partnership with local storekeeper Arthur Henderson, I took up the offer and increased the flock to 50 ewes.

The system called for adroit management for it was not an exercise in farming alone. When the ground was needed for rugby and other sports it was necessary to remove the sheep. That meant driving the flock along the main highway to my domestic acres. This was not a simple exercise for it entailed passing through the township and making an abrupt left turn at a busy road junction. The residents of Ohaeawai who seldom shut their gates, also frowned upon the prospect of a hungry flock devouring their flowers and vegetables. The hotel also had easy access to its backyard to which itinerant ovines would have been less than welcome. When circumstances demanded a change of pasture, as many helpers as possible had to be recruited. We owned no dog, many entrances needed to be blocked, and the road south had to be guarded lest the flock missed the left turn and continued on towards Pakaraka and further horizons.

Lambing time was also one of difficulty because it was necessary to have the ewes under close supervision. It was also the height of the rugby season so the main area of grazing was not available to them. Therefore we had to use our rather inadequate two acres.

From April to June the home paddocks were spelled and a carpet of mostly luxuriant kikuyu grass eventually covered the place. A couple of weeks before lambing was due to start we shifted the flock to where they had enough to eat. Armed with crook to catch the patients, I carried out observatory patrols as often as I could. Towards the end of lambing, feed started to get a bit short but a few blocks of concentrated molasses filled the gap until the rugby season ended. The flock, which had by now more than doubled, returned more slowly and with even more difficulty than before to the sports ground.

My farmer readers will no doubt have concluded that we were stocking pretty heavily and they would be right. However, we were also supplementing to achieve specific aims and were prepared to buy ourselves out of trouble. I was about to become involved in the phenomenon of heavy stocking on a far wider scale.

Towards the end of the 1950's and a bit beyond, much attention was focused on trials being carried out at the Ruakura Animal Research Station in relation to the stocking rates of dairy cows. The work was supervised and reported on by the talented Dr C.P. McMeekan, who showed that carrying capacity could be dramatically increased to a level producing 500 lbs of butterfat and beyond for each acre of pasture grazed. At that time the call was for higher production. The philosophy of higher stocking was taken up by government and its advisors, led by the then Minister of Agriculture. Unhappily, McMeekan's work was misinterpreted by many whose enthusiasm exceeded their intellect. Some thought that all they had to do to increase their wealth was to milk more cows, so skinny cows with amputated tails became the fashion.

Many farmers failed to note that McMeekan's outstanding results had been achieved with carefully bred cows, expertly milked and managed. Although stocked at 1.6 cows for each acre they were still averaging 308 lbs of butterfat per cow, much higher than the Northland average before the high stocking philosophy had been embraced. When some farmers increased their stocking rate their cow production in a number of cases fell to as low as 120 lbs of butterfat per cow. At times I was being called to attend animals clearly suffering from starvation. Their owners and sometimes advisors, mesmerised by the philosophy of high stocking, seemed unable to appreciate the situation.

A dairy cow needs a certain amount of tucker to keep her alive. If she is going to have a calf and produce a surplus, which is what the dairy farmer depends upon for his living, she needs a bit more. If uncontrolled increase in stocking takes place, clearly the point is reached where the cows only maintain themselves and have nothing left to provide income for their owners. If stocking rates are still increased, then the cows start to die or become highly vulnerable to the ravages of metabolic ills, like milk fever, grass staggers, or bacterial assault from organisms causing mastitis. McMeekan covered most of these points in his excellent book *Grass to Milk* which I consider one of the outstanding contributions to the New Zealand dairy industry. The book later formed a cornerstone on which my own farming philosophy was based. Unhappily the wide misinterpretation of

McMeekan's work cost farmers dearly and caused their animals much anguish.

The problem, which was unkindly called 'advisory disease' by some, was not only confined to dairy farms. The usually conservative sheep and beef farmers also wanted to get into the act and some bumped up their stock numbers, often with devastating results. Grass, short through heavy stocking, but fast growing as light and warmth increased in August, became very low in magnesium. This caused significant mortality in beef herds around calving. Sleepy sickness in ewes, a metabolic disturbance associated with low feed intake during the last month or so of pregnancy, and especially in ewes carrying twins, appeared to increase. It was a great time for vets but a trying one for the man on the land. It is important that those disposed to give advice have the expertise and integrity to do so.

About this time I acquired our first bit of farm land, 12 acres on one side of the road and another six on the other. This was a small block of stony, volcanic country near the Ohacawai township. It was at the junction where the Remuera Settlement Road — no relationship to its better-known and affluent Auckland counterpart — left Highway 12. The property had about two acres of grass, the remainder being covered in fern and gorse from which protruded the summits of large rocks at regular intervals.

A murmuring waterway meandered along the eastern boundary. Near the southern boundary it bubbled over a fairly wide expanse of flat rock before cascading into a deep and placid pool where eels lurked and local children loved to swim. The banks of this stream were an idyllic site for a dwelling and at that time it was our intention to so proceed. This however never happened, as ambition drove us to higher things and most likely wiser fortunes.

For now though, this new land needed a lot of attention. I had purchased a second-hand trailer and when time allowed it was hitched to the Landrover and used to move stones. These provided all-weather access from the road for the gateway became a muddy wallow when it rained. A bulldozer was engaged to shift the larger rocks into line, roughly bisecting the eastern part of the property and forming a substantial base for a rock wall of the future. The same machine pushed, pulled, harrowed and levelled — leaving an expanse of roughly even, dark volcanic soil. In autumn I sprinkled grass seed at the recommended rate. The result was spectacular and within a few weeks a healthy sole of verdant grass was established. It made farming look easy. I had yet to learn that the volcanic soil of the north could also propagate gorse, tobacco weed, ink weed and thistles at an astonishing rate. It was not until spring, still a few months away, that these aggressive plants showed their potential to convert the place to a wilderness even more weedy than it had been before.

Meanwhile, a local identity called Johnny Tubbs erected another fence in expert fashion despite the stones. This gave us three paddocks, and it would have been good business to introduce sheep at this point to closely graze and nip off burgeoning gorse plants as they emerged. However, the road and boundary fences were a long way off being sheep-proof. Instead I acquired half-a-dozen steers to fill the gap until I could upgrade the fences. The steers were a mixed bunch of 18-month-old cattle, mostly shorthorn but quiet enough. This was my first venture into cattle farming — and cattle rustling. Late one Saturday afternoon a farmer on the Remuera Road rang to say that on the way home from the rugby he had noticed some of my cattle on the roadside. Knowing that cattle on the road after dark posed a threat to life and limb, I climbed into the Landrover and sped off to investigate.

I passed the road gate of the property and found it was still shut, although a piece of fencing wire which I had introduced as an extra precaution had been unwound and was lying nearby. Half-a-mile up the road I came upon my cattle peacefully grazing the 'long acre'. Nearby were two children aged around nine and riding ponies. I naturally posed a question or two to these youthful equestrians before recovering my stock and returning them to their paddock. The children, with bland expression, explained that they were only passing, an assertion hard to dispute. Perhaps so, but how then did the cattle escape? One theory, later explained to me by one of experience in such matters, was that if I had not intervened, the stock would have been gently moved on as dusk fell. They would have found a new home in a paddock owned by friends or relatives of the mounted children. Perhaps yes, maybe no, but a mystery still unsolved. I now applied a chain and padlock to my gate and thereafter our cattle stayed where they were supposed to be.

I only owned this first farm for a little over a year and although others made progress with the place I was always a bit sorry that the plans for our Shangri-La were never brought to fruition.

Our First 'Real' Farm

It is surprising that after over 10 years of observing and often trying to correct the many trials and tribulations which farming seemed to attract, I should still feel an attraction for the land and its grazing stock. One reason was perhaps genealogical. Ever since Matthew Steel married Mary Mochrie in 1703, my mother's family had farmed the not always rewarding country of central Scotland. They continue to do so to this day, although I am pleased to say my cousin's present holding near Edinburgh looks far better than some of its predecessors.

There was another reason. Often when I told my clients to do this and not that in relation to their management practices, which had important impact on the veterinary situation on their farms, I would be met with a dismissive shrug. They would make the observation that if I was farming I would know that what I had just suggested was neither possible nor practical. I wanted to be part of this action and demonstrate that theory and practice could indeed be merged with advantage. I think my early perception, like in many things, was partly right and partly wrong. When I finally grasped the nettle and bit the bullet, I did indeed discover that the comments of my farmer clients had more than a modicum of truth in them.

Eric Baldwin, was a friend and mentor of long-standing. My erstwhile landlord and still client had continued our association in a professional sense and in other ways. We had jointly purchased a clinker-built dinghy with an eight horsepower vintage outboard motor. I can recall two things about it. One was a hole in the petrol tank over which someone had welded a sixpence as a suitable patch, and the other was the apparent absence of a clutch or, for most of the time, any control of the throttle. The result was that if and when the outboard started the vessel took off at high speed, threatening to propel its occupants into the sea. Despite these difficulties we had a number of successful fishing expeditions, and on one occasion I recall a delighted Eric landing a snapper weighing 23 pounds.

As often happens while waiting for the fish to bite, conversation turned to other things. Eric mentioned that if he could get a buyer he wouldn't mind shifting to a larger property further south. My pulse quickened — here was a chance. The farm was close to the township of Ohaeawai on Highway 1 and was thus an acceptable centre for my practice. But how? I had never been a great borrower and raising finance in that way was an option I never really considered, strange as that way of thinking may now seem. However, fate or whoever controls it, took a hand. Two events of significance came to pass almost within the hour. A local stock agent wanted to buy a centrally located property away from town and ours was just that. The indefatigable Arthur Henderson, storekeeper turned farmer, was now even more enthusiastic than before and was a ready buyer for our 18 acres. Eric wanted £17,000 for his farm and with the offers for our house and mini-farm plus a bit we had saved, there was just enough to launch the deal. It was all go.

Now that we had a farm the question was what to do with it. Eric was milking 80 cows on the 100 or so acres of cleared land with good results. It was really our intention to run sheep and cattle, but fences which adequately hold dairy cows do not necessarily contain smaller sheep and more aggressive cattle. As the farm had a long road frontage on Highway 1 I viewed the prospect of wandering stock being in frequent contact with passing traffic as a matter of concern. If we stuck with the cows, who was going to milk them? Hardly me, already heavily committed to matters veterinary. My wife perhaps — a not unusual arrangement in those days. I told her the story of one of my clients whose children from four to seven actively helped with the milking, while the younger ones of ages around one or two were deposited in cream cans in the cowshed to keep them out of mischief and machinery. At the same time the young ones gained first-hand knowledge of the tasks they would eventually be called upon to perform. The story was received with interest but not, in any way, as a blueprint for application in our case.

Again, fate intervened for it so happened that I had engaged a burly young German called Karl Marxen to cut down some large macrocarpa trees on our southern boundary. The idea was to convert the timber to posts for use on our new farm we were buying. The energy which Karl applied to his task quite astonished me. Although he didn't talk a lot, he did mention that marriage was an early objective but he was being frustrated by an inability to find suitable accommodation. Now Bill Low, then chairman of my board and interested in my latest endeavours, told me that the government was committed to promoting housing for farm employees as an impetus to increasing farm production. It made loans available to promote the construction of houses for farm workers. These 'suspensory loans' were cancelled and no repayment required if a farm employee occupied the dwelling for seven years. I put a proposition to Karl and another to the

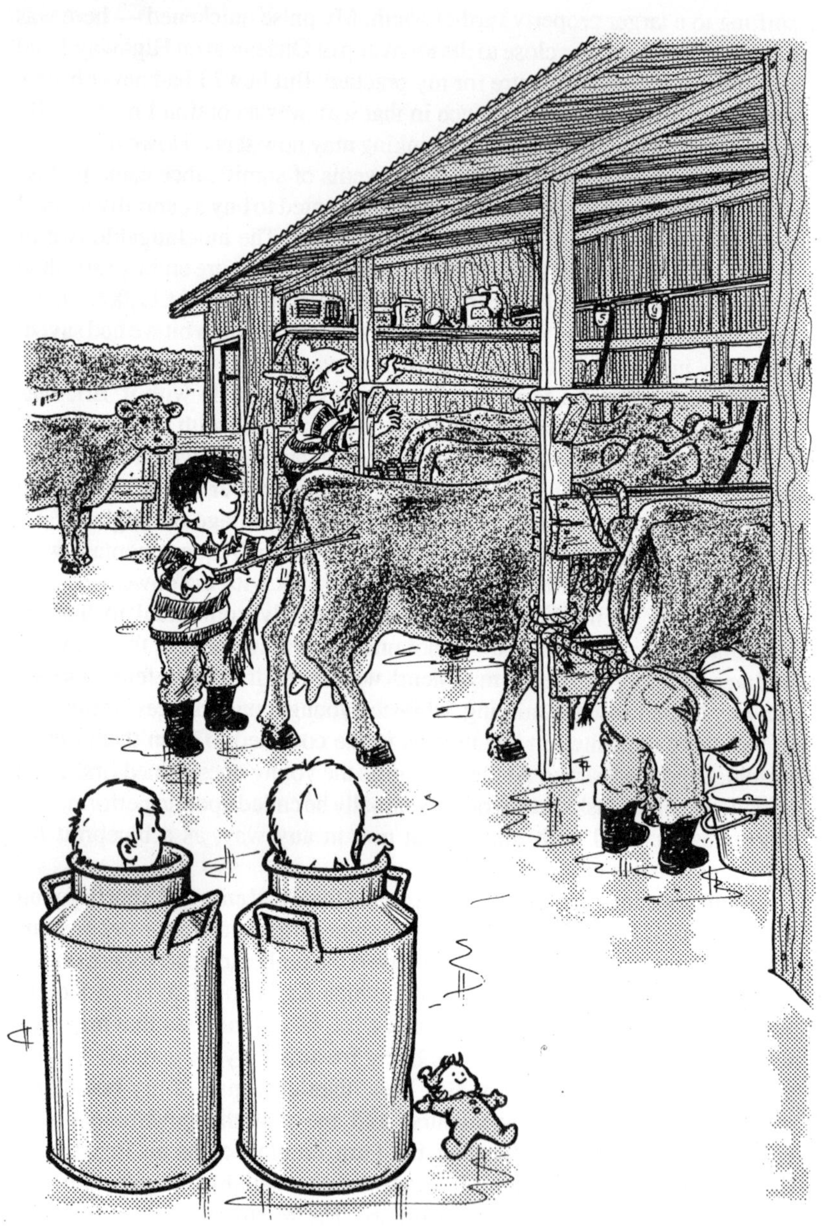

department which authorised the loan and both were successful. I now had a sharemilker engaged on a 39 percent basis but who had never milked a cow in his life. I also had the means whereby I could put a roof over his head. Intuition was perhaps more at work than judgement but at the end of the day it seemed to work.

As takeover day in May approached I set about buying surplus stock from my clients. As might be expected the herd was a mixed bunch, predominantly Jersey. It is always difficult to assemble a herd free from disease and of good productive capacity, unless purchased as a going concern. I was lucky in one respect for one member of the herd I assembled was a gentle Friesian, called Ellerlea Bonny Choice. She became our top producer and encouraged us to later form our Friesian stud of which she was the foundation matron. She proved to be a very bonny choice.

Finance for the milker's cottage soon came to hand and a start was made in its construction. It was sited near where the farm's boundary joined that of the Ohaeawai township, making it possible for the occupants of the cottage to walk to school, post office, garage, store and hotel, although the latter was never much of an attraction for the people who worked for me. Patience was not one of Karl's many virtues and as some of the cows were starting to look as if they would calve at any moment I too was concerned that we might soon have a lactating herd without anyone to milk them. However, we just made it and Karl and his new wife took up residence almost to the day when our first Jersey dropped her calf. And, as if determined to make use of the resident vet, she promptly developed milk fever. Luckily it was detected early and successfully treated.

It is always a wrench to leave a home and, as it was the first one we had established and lived in for over ten years, our departure proved no exception. It did give satisfaction though to reflect that we had most likely rescued the old place from oblivion and left it much better than we had found it, an important philosophical as well as practical objective. The tui still sang in the strawberry tree but this time the song was one of farewell.

We still visit our first home, now well over 100-years old, and it is pleasing to find it in good repair and occupied by an old friend who called the place *Linger Longer*. As I drove the Landrover and trailer crammed with the paraphernalia of domestic life up the drive and down the mile or so of road to our second home, I felt our new adventurous decision along paths as yet unknown, was right.

I had inherited a few sows and a boar from Eric Baldwin, but with only 60 cows, the farm was clearly understocked. I bought 90 wethers but the small paddock round the cowshed was the only one with sheep-proof fences. It was obvious that fencing was going to be a number one priority.

Fortunately, sharemilker Karl had the will and muscle to cope and soon things improved to the point where a few Angus steers could be added to control the burgeoning sea of grass.

The total area of our new farm was 155 acres, but around 50 acres were steep hills of clay at the back of the farm and covered in gorse. They were divided by two parallel clefts bordered by puriri trees whose hardwood timber had long been popular for use as fence posts. Maori legend had it that the puriris of Taiamai, of which the ones on our farm were part, laughed in delight but never in scorn. They laughed especially when some happy event like the restoration of peace or a visit from an eminent person was imminent. I heard them neither laugh nor cry when we took over — perhaps they were going to wait and see!

The eastern end of the range had been occupied by the Maoris of years gone and they had formed a pa. The terraced steps, although covered in gorse, were clearly evident.

There were a few paddocks near the road from which the rock had been cleared and the stone stacked neatly nearby, but for the most part rocky outcrops were evident and scattered boulders gave evidence of a tempestuous past. A stream tumbled in confusion over rocky outcrops, and at others times it proceeded more placidly below canopies of willow, totara and puriri. Near the eastern boundary where the stream finally took its leave, it formed a large pool where our children and those of our Maori neighbour loved to swim.

At the other end of the property just above the cowshed, a concrete dam had been constructed. Remnants of machinery also lay about. This had once generated electric power for the adjacent cowshed, as well as for two houses and the Ohaeawai hall.

The house on the farm was fairly basic although the Baldwins had added a new bedroom and a garage. There was about an acre of tree-dotted lawn and although I had purchased a large rotary petrol-driven mower it still took over two hours to cope with the prolific growth. Luckily it was winter but I determined that before the grass explosion of spring took place there would need to be a few changes — like using sheep as lawn mowers.

A more urgent problem was the provision of a surgery. My board agreed to pay me a rental and I borrowed £250 from them, the rent received being roughly equivalent to the interest attracted. Carpenter Billy Woods was still around and he soon boarded up the front of the garage and lined the inside with hardboard. A stainless steel sink and the 'Zip' heater I had recovered from my old surgery were soon installed and some shelves and cupboards completed the transformation. As I now had space, I persuaded my board — now more sympathetic to the pet owners of the district — to supply a much larger operating table. It was not too long before the shelves and cupboards were stocked with the medicines and appliances I needed. Then I awaited the arrival of the cats and dogs, birds and rabbits.

The family vehicles were doing it a bit hard though, for the garage was no longer fulfilling its original function. The Landrover was no problem for it was used to standing outside, and worse. But the Consul we had been given in Scotland was more sensitive. The old tractor shed at the back of the house was quite waterproof but could only be reached through the paddock. In winter it did not provide a surface the car's tyres could easily grip. The Landrover was usually able to encourage the stranded car on its way, but my wife had to negotiate her return to the house through the muddy paddock in footwear designed for paved walkways. She wasn't particularly happy.

As June moved into July more cows calved and the chug of the separator in the cowshed at last indicated that we were in business. I think Karl must have taken a crash course in milking somewhere for he seemed to be managing pretty well, even if a bit unorthodox at times. I had gone to a clearing sale at Opua and bought a secondhand Ferguson 24 tractor which I drove home through town and country. This was the first time I had driven a tractor, although I had often been a passenger. I was sometimes left wondering how I survived. On one occasion I was a passenger in another Ferguson when the farmer driver, anxious to expedite treatment to his bloated cows, charged down the sloping bank of a stream and up the other side. With the threat of being deposited between the fast-moving wheels of the tractor, I clasped my client round the neck in a desperate but successful attempt to avoid mutilation.

The one aspect of farming over which I felt I had least control was the pig side, particularly with regard to the pregnant sows and their lord and master the boar. The sows were allowed free range, roaming over the farm and subsisting on a diet of grass alone until they farrowed. They were supposedly meant to be then confined in the piggery where they and their fast-growing offspring could be fed a diet of skim milk until the youngsters were weaned at about six weeks of age. The mother was then returned to the great outdoors to await the attention of the boar. The cohabitation resulted in the production of another litter hopefully before Christmas when there was still enough skim milk being produced to sustain it.

It was not always easy to predict when the sows were going to farrow, although it always seemed to happen when the weather was at its worst. I had been watching the black sow with a white stripe round her middle for a day or so. She had developed the habit of coming up to the back gate each evening for the bountiful supply of household scraps. One wet and windy night there was no sign of Scraps as we had called her. Investigation found her rooting up fern and grass in a corner of the orchard a few hundred yards or so across the paddock from the house. Clearly, as sows do, she was preparing a bed indicating that farrowing was imminent, with the weather turning rough and something of a gale blowing out of the north-east.

Down the garden path from our dwelling was a disused fowl house. If Scraps could be induced to take up residence there, the happy event could take place in circumstances more congenial than what she herself planned. Mustering such domestic help as was available, with homework forgotten and dinner placed on hold, we cajoled the protesting pig across the paddock. Bribed by a trail of scraps and with periodic prods from behind, she at last entered her new home. I secured the door by sliding a piece of inch pipe through a couple of staples provided for the purpose.

Ever the perfectionist, and knowing that warmth was a necessity for the survival of newborn piglets, I strung a long flex lead from a plug in the wash-house. The other end I connected to a heat lamp which I had previously used to treat a bruised shoulder, sustained when I fell over the rail in a cowshed, trying to escape an angry bull who failed to appreciate the efforts I was making on his behalf.

After half-an-hour or so, a peep through a crack in the door revealed a reclining Scraps grunting happily. Twenty minutes later the numbers in the erstwhile farrowing house had increased to three. Close to midnight when most of the exhausted family had gone to bed, the numbers of piglets had increased to fourteen. At last the mother and myself appropriately called it a day. I did not expect such a large porcine family to survive, but in the end she reared nine, so our efforts had not been in vain.

Although the problem of sows farrowing wherever they fancied was one which concerned me, it was surprising how efficient these mothers were in selecting their place of confinement. Often a matron, missing for awhile, would turn up grazing the abundant autumn-saved pasture, with half-a-dozen or more piglets tailing along behind. The choice of pregnant pigs was, as far as a place to farrow was concerned, sometimes selfish. Jack Abbott, my young assistant who had newly arrived from the south of Scotland, was living in a caravan behind our house until he could find somewhere more permanent. In his spare time Jack was very much a man of the sea and he had been constructing a runabout in an old shed behind our house. One morning he was most surprised to find a litter of eight and their mother comfortably installed in a nest of tarpaulins, life jackets, rainproof gear, and other things that boaties use. It was typical porcine opportunism!

In the meantime, it was most likely safer for sows to farrow where they could. Unless properly constructed farrowing pens were provided it was inevitable that many young pigs would be crushed between the unyielding concrete of walls and floor and the ponderous bulk of their mother. She was usually too clumsy to avoid her numerous charges all the time. During the first year on the farm I constructed two proper farrowing pens, with guard rails low down round the walls. They proved useful, although they took away something of the drama and excitement which the free-range sows provided from time to time.

Our farm had an undoubted location value because it stretched along the main road for about a mile. However this exposed most of the farm and its operation to all who passed by and that included a fair proportion of my clients. During the first spring one of our Jersey cows indulged herself in the clover-rich pasture and succumbed to bloat. This was a common and often rapidly fatal condition due to excessive gas production in the commodious first stomach. Unfortunately, this fatality took place in a paddock near the road and although my man had the carcase speedily removed and buried in an old creek bed we had reserved as a cemetery, it was just surprising how many had noted the fatality.

'See you had a dead cow the other day,' was the knowing greeting I often received for a week or two. Remarks about how much feed we had or didn't have were frequent and it soon became clear to me that the district was now passing a dual judgement on me — my performance in the field as a vet and my performance in the paddock as a farmer.

The first season drifted on and we were lucky that no floods, droughts or other catastrophes intervened. I did learn however, that the peaceful stream below the cowshed could quite quickly become a raging torrent if heavy rain fell. This was no great problem for I had been arranging the fences so that as few as possible crossed the creek, thus minimising repair work when flood carried all before it. If the flood came suddenly or at night there was a different sort of difficulty. If the cows happened to be on the opposite side of the creek from the cowshed, they literally had to swim for their milking. It was an adventure which seemed a lot less of concern to them than to me, watching their progress with heads only showing above the torrent and visualising our hard-won herd ending up battered over waterfalls or entangled in wire or willows downstream.

As Christmas 1961 came and went I began to feel more in control, although all the time I was a non-milking dairy farmer it was always a concern that I was dependent on others to milk the cows. There are few tasks more demanding. Morning and night the cows were always there. In this respect I think that I was luckier than most and as the dairy season started on its downward curve it became clear that the scratch herd of 60 milked by a milker who had never milked before, was going to produce a bit over 18,000 lbs of butter fat. Although it was 4,000 lbs less than what Eric had achieved on the same property, he had used 80 cows. We had also been carrying around 30 beef cattle plus a few wethers. I thought the situation encouraging and not too bad for a beginner. I had a concern of a different sort for my aging father in Scotland. He had not followed up the arrangements I had made for him to follow us and his letters were few. I knew that two of my aunts had died and felt that despite pressure of practice and the farm I had an obligation to return to Scotland.

Sojourn to Scotland

In those days no large jet planes came to New Zealand and it was necessary to join the fast Sydney-San Francisco service at Nandi in Fiji. I left from Whenuapai in a jet-prop aircraft operated by Tasman Empire Airways. After a stop of several hours at San Francisco, I headed across America by B.O.A.C. After nearly a day's wait in New York, a fairly slow trip across the Atlantic in a B.O.A.C. Britannia aircraft finally set me down at Prestwick in Scotland. It was a journey of length but little leisure, which would have been well suited to anyone doing research into jet lag and related disorders.

The trip had important repercussions for me in another way for among the expectant passengers at Whenuapai I recognised John Duncan, a well-known Wellington businessman who represented the New Zealand Kennel Club on the National Hydatids Council. John was travelling alone on business to London and suggested that I might like to join him for dinner in San Francisco where we would have some time to wait for our connecting flight. As John was travelling first-class and I — in keeping with my more modest means — was seated towards the tail of the aircraft, I did not see much of him until we met in the busy concourse of the San Francisco airport.

True to his promise, John soon hailed a taxi and we sped along the multi-lane highway towards the centre of the city. Our destination was the well-known Mark Hopkins Hotel. This hotel was a famous rendezvous and the view from the bar at the Top of the Mark that evening was as outstanding as any city landscape anywhere. The sparkling harbour with its Golden Gate Bridge held the eye, with the sombre Alcatraz a reminder, even in that backdrop of beauty, of the weakness of man. As the day faded into the mists of evening the city lights took over to display a different panorama indicating that nature was not alone in her artistry.

After a few rounds of drinks and a few of the bar — literally, for it was a revolving one — we descended to one of the restaurants. The decor was of green Hunting Stewart tartan and here we enjoyed what I supposed was about the best cuisine America could offer. Despite our fatigue, conversation soon became more expansive. John told me that he owned a third share in a farm at Waimate North and he was concerned about its management. He was too far away in Wellington to be of any practical use, while another partner also did not live near at hand. The third owner, on whose shoulders rested most of the responsibility, was quite elderly and although he lived reasonably close he was in indifferent health. John wondered if I knew the farm and could comment on it. I said I was aware of the place although my professional attendances had been few and this was usually a sign of very good or very bad management.

'What say,' said John after a bit of reflection, 'that I buy out my partners and you supervise the place for me?'

I have always made it a rule never to give firm commitments in a social environment and none could have been more social than where I was then, so I said I would think about it when I returned to New Zealand. This I did, and after a further approach by John I took up his suggestion with implications I will later relate.

Later that night we flew on across America, and from New York John left for London while I headed for Scotland.

I spent a bit over a month in Scotland renewing old acquaintance with people and places. For the most part they were still as I remembered them, although a few high rises were starting to dominate the skylines while the River Clyde was clearly losing its industrial dominance. The National Hydatids Council had asked me to make some investigations into some aspects of the diseases with which it was concerned and I visited a few pet food establishments, abattoirs and the veterinary faculty of Liverpool University. I made one or two interesting discoveries. The disease was practically non-existent in Scotland, mainly because farm dogs — perhaps like some of their owners — were fed mainly porridge, bread, milk and biscuits. Offal was used to manufacture food for people (haggis perhaps?). In Wales however, the dogs were more generously treated. Sometimes they became infected with the parasite although nothing like the extent experienced in New Zealand. The pet food establishments I visited were quite sophisticated with white coats, tea and biscuits being provided for visitors who were clearly viewed as potential customers. I discovered that quite a proportion of the raw material for these establishments came from New Zealand, having been rejected there for one reason or another — mostly hydatid and other parasites. Fortunately they could not survive the process of freezing for preservation and the subsequent cooking used in the preparation of pet food.

It was pointed out to me that the livers imported for pet food were mostly in better shape than those sold in Britain for human consumption. In Britain the presence of another parasitic disease caused by liver fluke made it difficult to find a liver not in some way affected by this ubiquitous parasite. Butchers, realising that livers with traces of fluke would have little aesthetic appeal, sometimes made a habit of displaying the offal, thinly sliced and angled on a tray, so providing a degree of camouflage enhanced with a bit of parsley on top for good measure. A trick of the trade I surmised. It also sometimes happened that the New Zealand product which was supposed to be used for pet food was adjudged far too good for that, and illegally found its way into the human food chain. One shrewd pet food manager hinted that perhaps he should not be extending such hospitality to me, for if New Zealand was successful in eliminating hydatids and like parasites, his main source of high-class raw material for his pet food enterprise would disappear. The ill wind of the parable apparently was working well in his favour.

I also discovered that in Britain the horse sometimes exhibited hydatid cysts although of a rather different type from that involving sheep and cattle. As far as I knew, equines in New Zealand were not involved.

On my return to New Zealand I prepared a report for the National Hydatids Council which at that time was very interested in the subject of cooked dog foods as a possible alternative to the raw meat and offal being widely fed and at the bottom of the whole problem. I did in fact conduct some experiments with a block-type, high-fat ration prepared in cooperation with Des Cochrane, a butcher in the Bay of Islands. I later cooperated with a Wanganui firm which produced a dog sausage. After a few false and sometimes odiferous starts owing to poor shelf life, the dog sausage achieved a degree of acceptability and is indeed commercially produced and marketed to this day.

But I get ahead. I flew out of Heathrow on a flight to Nandi but engine trouble in New York and an unscheduled delay at Honolulu left me feeling much like a competitor in the Grand National must feel after completing the course. I slept the clock round in the Star Hotel, picked up a new Landrover and headed home to family, farm and friends.

The Deadly Disease

In the first half of the 1960's there was considerable debate concerning the introduction of a scheme to control bovine tuberculosis, a disease dating back to biblical times. It had been established in New Zealand for many years after having no doubt been introduced with injudicious imports from countries such as Britain where the disease had flourished for even longer. Of course, in earlier times there was no test to indicate symptomless carriers, so little blame can be attached to the settlers of that era.

The significance of the disease was threefold. In the first place it caused serious losses in cattle, especially dairy cows. It was the main condition on which world-wide meat inspection methods were based. Pigs were often involved through being fed tuberculous skim milk. The disease was also important because the bovine strain, although slightly different from its human counterpart, could easily be spread to people. Children were particularly susceptible because they were often given raw milk to drink. In Britain, most of the bone and joint manifestations of the disease involved children and were of bovine origin. Another emerging reason to control the disease was that our main customers had schemes in place to eliminate tuberculosis from their herds, and there was pressure for New Zealand to take similar steps.

The disease was most often acquired through contaminated drinking water or maybe eating pasture grazed by already infected stock. It was often first evident as white or creamy cheese-like lesions in the lymphatic glands draining the intestines. Depending on the resistance of the afflicted animal, it could rapidly spread. More often its spread was insidious, taking years to significantly progress and involving any or all of the vital organs, especially the glands of the head, the liver and lungs. Coughing further spread the bacteria to pasture and to the water in troughs or in ponds where they lingered because there was no continuous flow to flush them away. The few farmers who visited the works to see their infected stock slaughtered were often horrified at the depredation the disease had made in animals they thought to be healthy.

While still a student in Scotland I had been involved in the early efforts to eliminate tuberculosis. Looking back, I must say that the method adopted then was indeed ponderous and relatively inefficient. Animals that had reacted to the test were actually allowed to be marketed, although in a special ring in the markets. Milk was labelled according to the herd of its origin, with produce from tuberculosis-free herds sold at a higher price, ensuring that the less wealthy had a better chance of becoming infected. Class distinction indeed!

The test for tuberculosis involved the injection within the skin of a small amount of tuberculin, a sterile product from the artificial culture of the bacteria. If the cow had tuberculosis it usually exhibited an allergic reaction in the form of a swelling which was measured by callipers. A description of the swelling was recorded on large forms, and sent to the Ministry of Agriculture for their evaluation. It was soon found that cattle were sometimes infected with harmless bird tuberculosis and they too sometimes reacted to the test. To distinguish the two an injection of avian Tuberculin was also given at the same time. If a cow reacted to both bovine and avian types the result was disregarded and a re-test scheduled. The injections were given on the side of the neck and I recall often dodging the long horns of Ayrshire cattle doing their best to discourage people with sharp syringes from carrying out the tests they had to perform.

In New Zealand, 20 or so years on, the approach was to be more direct with compulsory slaughter of reactors. A single injection of Tuberculin was injected within the skin of one of the two folds below the bovine tail — an easier place to get at than, for instance, the neck. Interpretation was to depend on the visual and tactile skill of the tester which, even if it was a bit like an umpire giving a l.b.w. decision at cricket, it had the merit of simplicity. With a bit of practice, it was a skill easily acquired.

Sometimes when I hesitated when reading a test the look of concern or anguish which crossed my client's face gave an indication of an emotional battle within. Despite the adequate compensation paid, the true man of the land did not take lightly to losing a member of the family, so to speak, or the knowledge that a deep-seated problem might be on the verge of threatening his enterprise.

However, the New Zealand system failed to recognise some of the problems which had been well documented overseas, such as the difficulties associated with avian infection. While avian tuberculosis was never a problem here, there was a condition which was, especially in the northern half of the North Island. The harmless, so-called skin tuberculosis was caused by an organism which looked like the real thing but caused only lumps in the skin. It irregularly caused a reaction to the tuberculin test. Even after a test had been carried out this skin infection remained in the herd, ready to cause continuing problems. This meant that some cattle were being slaughtered without being infected with tuberculosis. When no evidence of this disease was apparent during the post mortem the concern of their owners was understandable. Various alternative check tests were later devised which may have helped to sort out the problem, but just the same I think quite a few clean cattle were killed.

The testing programme fell mainly on the practicing members of the veterinary profession. This was a considerable extra workload which had to be carried out mainly when the cows were dry, as farmers did not want the herd upset and reactors removed when it was in full production. This fitted in fairly well, for early winter was the quietest time of the year. Dairy cows were easy to handle although walking, tight-rope fashion, along the platform of a herringbone cowshed with syringe in hand was not the easiest of exercises. Self-injection with Tuberculin could cause a painful local and sometimes unpleasant general reaction.

Young stock and eventually beef cattle were different propositions and the mud of winter helped not at all. The traumatic input on the operator was twofold for the quickest way to test was to have the subjects crushed closely together and move through the restless throng, syringe in one hand and a stick of raddle chalk in the other with which to identify the treated animals. Steel toe-caps saved the toes, but by the end of a testing day the rest of the feet often looked a bit blue. Races were supposed to be provided for stock to be tested, and they often were, but in many cases they were too high. With the traffic of stock over the muddy floor, the sinking stock retreated more and more out of reach as time went on. Suspended jack-knife style over the top rail of a race, administering to stock far below, gave one a heady feeling and a fair amount of contusion below the rib cage and maybe even what lay below that.

One result of the testing programme was that I ventured to places I had not before seen, for while it was never compulsory to call the vet the stock owners were compelled by statute to submit their stock for testing. One such place was reached by a pendulous bridge of timber and fencing wire strung between two totaras above a raging torrent swollen by the rains of winter. The farmers were bachelor brothers, and rather odd characters at that. They owned a small house and a large bulldozer whose value I estimated would have exceeded that of the farm and stock combined. The bulldozer was apparently used as a general work horse for, as I approached the cowshed I could see it approaching down a steep track in the gorse-covered hills. Its wide blade shepherded a motley collection of stock of all sizes, shape, sex and age — a method of mustering I had not seen before.

The Department of Agriculture had a fair idea where most of the dairy farms were, because they were able to obtain such information from the dairy factory which for the most part knew where its suppliers lived. Sometimes however, when testing a Maori herd out in the back-blocks, I could identify further mobs of cattle away on the horizon being driven along roads and tracks never identified on any map. Relatives and friends had heard the vet was coming to test, and for social as well as veterinary reasons wanted to get in on the act. Although I had no authority, I used to test such itinerant mobs as well. Otherwise the programme might well have passed them by and who could tell what problems these mavericks concealed?

Despite a few hiccups the scheme to control bovine tuberculosis advanced, and by the end of the sixties the disease was well on its way to near elimination. Sadly, in recent times there is evidence that it is being revived largely because of the rapid increase in the numbers of opossums. The opossums are uncontrolled carriers of the disease, highly susceptible to tuberculosis and picking it up through their close association with each other and then contaminating pastures on which cattle graze. In the time of which I mainly write, opossums had not established themselves and were not therefore a complicating factor. I hope that the efforts made by many and the heartbreak endured by a few, may not have been in vain and efforts will soon be vigorously made to control this unpleasant immigrant. It threatens not only our major pastoral industry but a wide variety of plant and fauna for which this land is rightly renowned.

The practice was now busier than ever with the tuberculosis testing programme an additional load. With two colleagues in Kaikohe and Jack Abbott now installed at Kerikeri, I had managed to contract my personal responsibility to the area of Ohaeawai and Waimate North together with Kawakawa. This cut down my travelling obligations considerably, although holidays and sickness in the rest of the team meant visits elsewhere from time to time. There were also other inroads into my time. The farm did not occupy me much in an active role as I always had a manager. My function was chiefly that of administrator and decision maker. I was soon to become involved in another farm management situation, for John Duncan had followed up his proposal made to me in San Francisco and bought out his partners at *Northlands* at Waimate North. I was also involved with my membership of the National Hydatids Council and this meant an absence of a day or two each month in Wellington or somewhere else.

I began to sense that one or two members of my board felt my interests had spread too widely than was usual for what, after all, was a dairy company employee, especially as I was now a shareholder in the major company which employed me. This is not unusual nowadays but it was frowned upon then. I did not feel that the work for which I was paid was being unduly compromised, but I had never been a fan of the club system and would have preferred a more personal client-vet relationship which private practice ensured. But it was then that an opportunity came my way from the unlikely source of the United States of America. The U.S.A. had made it one of the conditions of the export of meat to them that vets be stationed in freezing works supplying the meat. As there were few vets in New Zealand who were interested in this type of employment full-time, part-time work was offered on a half-day basis plus mileage. I indicated my interest in the large Moerewa plant only 10 miles down the road and was told that if I applied I would most likely get the job.

So far so good, but in the terms of my contract with my board I was only able to start in private practice with its permission if the area covered by my proposed practice coincided with any area it serviced.

'You'll starve,' said the chairman. 'Go to it,' said the board. The canny Scot in me told me that I was now in quite a satisfactory situation. Whatever happened in the clinical practice my work at Moerewa would underpin it financially. With two children at boarding school and a farm inclined to take rather more than it gave, this was quite important. Then I had another piece of good fortune. The burgeoning scheme to control bovine tuberculosis was in place and the Department of Agriculture was in something of a quandary. The testing allocation had previously been given to the club and not personally to me, although I had carried out a significant part of the testing. In the end, in what I think was a good decision, the Department decided to ask the farmers involved who they wanted to do their testing. I received 90 percent support, and on this basis I was allocated the whole area in which I had personally practiced — a total of 27,000 head to be tested — a welcome support for the new venture, but implying a lot of hard work. It is always rewarding to serve and, one way or the other, make things better than before. Although the club system did not give me the independence I sought, without it I most likely would never have come here at all.

The Major Industry

My earliest connection with the meat industry was the same as that of many other members of the public, who with wrinkled nose and caustic comment passed the malodourous Moerewa freezing works.

The meat industry, sustained by the introduction of refrigeration and a stable market in the Old Country, was one of comfortable, slumbering affluence. Farmers, to their later sorrow, were mostly concerned with green pastures on which lambs gambolled and contented cattle grazed. When the trucks loaded with the end product of farming endeavour rolled off the farm, the average man on the land was less than familiar with their future. He was happy enough for things to stay that way. A mental block seemed to operate at the farm gate and eyes were turned again inwards towards the far more familiar and pleasant pastoral scene.

In the 1920's most of the plants were relatively new and there was a system of solo butchering. One man was responsible for the handling of each carcase in order to encourage high performance in the individual. Any misdemeanour relating to hygiene or anything else could at once be traced to its source. On the introduction of the chain system one operator usually performed one task and digressions could be concealed or diluted by the anonymity of numbers.

A government meat inspection system had long been in place but this was chiefly aimed at the detection of animal disease like bovine tuberculosis. Pigs also had their fair share of problems because they were being infected by tuberculous milk and also had a number of respiratory, intestinal and skin conditions as a result of inadequate diet and housing. Sheep had few problems of veterinary or public health significance. New Zealand's chief meat export to Britain was lamb. Britain's standards of inspection and meat hygiene were relatively primitive while freezing en route minimised much bacterial proliferation. New Zealand's standard lamb carcase was of a size ideally suited to the British table and it was much in demand.

But things in the major industry were about to change. I guess the catalyst was two-fold. It was clear that British entry into the European Community was sooner or later going to abolish Commonwealth preference in trade at least, and New Zealand's marketing strategy was in for a change. Another very important factor was the fast growing trade in beef for the American hamburger market. This ubiquitous sandwich needs an input of lean beef with a binding quality to blend with the more fatty domestic product. The New Zealand cull dairy cow and, more especially bull, provided the ideal constituent and an impressive trade soon built up which persists to this day.

The expansion of the American market triggered a series of events which were to have a profound, traumatic and expensive impact on the New Zealand scene, albeit also a very profitable one.

In America last century there was a close relationship between farmer, butcher and consumer. If the customer was dissatisfied there was quick complaint to the butcher who soon referred it to the farm of origin if that was where the substance of the shortcoming lay. This was most likely a fairly satisfactory situation. However, a disease like trichinosis was prevalent in pigs but invisible to the naked eye. It could be passed on to consumers without their knowledge.

As cities grew, the number of customers who wanted meat increased well beyond the capacity of local farmers to produce. Stock had to be brought from further afield and a new middle man in the form of large slaughtering plants evolved. The consumer lost direct influence and complaints, if any, where diluted by distance. The slaughtering plants, of which the ones in Chicago were the biggest, had high profit motives but few others, and so conditions soon deteriorated. Towards the end of the 19th century there was only limited meat inspection carried out. Usually it was at the behest of foreign customers importing American meat in which they sometimes found disturbing deviations from the normal. This was enough to establish a consumer prompted philosophy which half a century later was to have important repercussions in New Zealand.

By the turn of the century conditions in the American plants had become so bad that in 1906 President Theodore Roosevelt appointed a special committee of Charles P. Neill and James Bronson Reynolds to report. The report, which mainly covered the situation in Chicago after a surveillance of only two-and-a-half weeks, was damning in the extreme. They found odiferous toilets for both men and women situated close to working areas, high incidence of tuberculosis in workers, wooden floors left unclean and left saturated with blood and grease, aprons apparently seldom washed, and poor lighting and ventilation.

I quote: *'Workers toil without relief in a humid atmosphere heavy with odours of rotten wood, decayed meats, stinking offals and entrails — meat, sometimes old, recovered from dirt floors plus miscellaneous items like rope and pigskin and shovelled into current production, ultimately bearing the legend "The contents of this package have been inspected according to the Act of Congress of March 3, 1891 — Quality Guaranteed".'*

It was enough to upset the President and Congress and as a result they passed the Meat Inspection Act of 1906. This set standards of inspection, plant construction and maintenance as well as labelling of product. At this time the veterinary profession in America, unlike its counterparts in Britain and in New Zealand, took an active part in the developing situation. The American Veterinary Medical Association produced a comprehensive report relating to pending legislation. In this report, much of which seems to have been adopted, it was significant that it was recommended that progress be made under 'veterinary planning'. In the subsequent legislation the veterinary profession gained important statutory control of important aspects of the American meat industry including inspection, plant design and operation, labelling of product and so on. Later it was decided that the many countries wanting to export meat to America, needed to have a system comparable to that maintained by the American Federal Meat Inspection. This edict did not assert that all U.S. domestic plants so complied but it was as they say, the crunch for New Zealand.

To ensure that required standards were met, U.S. Department of Agriculture appointed officers who were veterinarians and were resident in the countries to which they had been allocated. I must say that I found these colleagues from over the sea, courteous and realistic in their outlook although I took some issue with some of their terms of reference. For instance, a system of control was required in New Zealand comparable with that operated by the Federal Meat Inspection. This was variously interpreted as 'the same as' or 'at least equal to'. This seemed fair enough but, hang on, there's a number of diseases in animals widespread in the United States but they don't occur here at all or, if they do, to such an extent as to made their implication of no consequence. So why carry out inspections, sometimes at high cost, specifically designed to discover diseases which are not there?

Beef measles and trichinosis are two good examples. Examination for beef measles could take up to 20 percent of beef inspection time and the latter needed the installation of expensive machines and people to operate them. The American requirements seemed to me to lack flexibility and remove discretion from their inspectors, thus devaluing their professional status to some extent.

Another rather odd point about the American approach was that there, inspectors seldom showed much interest about what happened in freezer stores. They also showed little interest in the products stored inside the stores. Failure of refrigerating machinery was by no means unusual and could lead to quite serious deterioration in product.

When it came to other parts of the plant things were different. I doubt if any New Zealand plant had reached the giddy depths of Chicago 1906 but this was 60 years on and our plants had time to mature. Some departments must have been at least equal to, the state of their American counterparts of long before. It was not surprising then that the American vets had a field day which lasted for a number of years. Flaking paint, rusty beams, cracked concrete, dripping chillers, smoking operators, wooden walls, roving rats, flies and cockroaches were all given the thumbs down. The great clean-up in the New Zealand meat industry had begun. Many will say not before time.

The U.S. Department of Agriculture was not yet finished. It announced that its officials would only talk and negotiate with their New Zealand opposites. This meant of course that the Americans wanted to consult only with the New Zealand Department of Agriculture and not with a multiplicity of meat companies and other organisations. This greatly simplified the approach from an American point of view. It also overcame embarrassing situations such as occurred in one South American country. An armed guard had to be placed at the hotel room door of a review officer to prevent unwelcome intrusion by friends or employees of the management of a local plant which had been downgraded.

In effect this meant a vet to vet dialogue and it also made it obligatory for a veterinary presence in all New Zealand export plants. The vets were also responsible for compliance with the American standards. This was certainly a challenge, especially as nearly all New Zealand vets regarded themselves as saviours of life rather than presidents of death. New outlook and new training would be needed if the new opportunities presented to the profession on a plate were to be seized.

Alas, the opportunity was not seen as such by the clinically orientated profession. It was still driven by its British tradition and full-time recruits for the many new jobs offering were few. The gap was filled by part-timers like myself, with mild inclination and still less competence. American graduates showed little interest but quite a number from various European countries were keen to immigrate. Despite some technical experience in the field some had doubtful academic qualifications and considerable language difficulty. One told me that on recruitment he had been told that English was spoken in freezing works but when he got here he found that that was not always so. Another, who was for the time being my boss, suggested that I conduct the American reviewer round the plant as it was a language he did not speak!

It was the part-timers like myself who bore the brunt of the early American intervention. The New Zealand Department of Agriculture was, I believe, wrong in its perception of the situation. It expected its veterinarians, most of whom lacked experience in this field, to administer detail of plant procedure and performance. The professional veterinarian should have confined his activities to surveillance and, if appropriate, certification that the product met the criteria laid down. However, plant vets became something of the meat in the sandwich and something of a club sandwich at that. We became embroiled in debate and argument over differing facets with the unions, lay meat inspectors, American reviewers, plant management, and even sometimes outsiders like contractors, truck drivers and angry farmers. It meant stopping production chains and attaching labels to dirty equipment in an effort to make management perform, so that the product it wanted to sell would merit certification.

All this fell within the lot of the plant veterinarian who must have felt that he was shooting himself in the foot most of the time. It was not surprising that the Government was trying to recruit from faraway places. There was also a rapid and dramatic increase in lay meat inspector numbers. This was because of the the lack of vets and also to inaugurate and supervise sometimes complicated systems of quality control so that management could be coerced into maintaining its product at the standard required.

I had many friends among meat inspectors. Although well-paid they carried out a repetitive job under unpleasant conditions with diligence. Perhaps I was fortunate, because relations between vets and meat inspectors were apparently not always amicable.

It is not surprising that many inefficiencies arose around this time as the different organisations involved assessed the developing situation and the role they had to play. The unions, ever perceptive, were perhaps first off the mark and were prepared to meet changes to technique and even manning if adequate financial rewards were forthcoming. Innovations like hand washing were welcomed if bracketed with monetary adjustment. Chants of 'hygiene, hygiene' were common on the dressing floors when a satisfactory financial or manning reward had failed to be negotiated.

Of the other players, management appeared mesmerised by what was happening. They seemed to regard American reviewing vets as some sort of visitors from outerspace (their hats certainly sometimes gave that impression!) possessing magical qualities of perception and pronouncement. Farming organisations and farmers, who in the end were going to have to foot the bill, took only a journalistic interest. As I have said before the man on the land was not overly keen in pursuing the future of his stock beyond the farm gate.

There therefore existed unions and reviewers who knew exactly what they wanted, for they had travelled such paths before, and a department and management floundering in new and troubled waters. It surprised me to see so many with the same declared objectives apparently proceeding in different directions.

I am far from denouncing the U.S. Department of Agriculture. As history shows it had seen it all before and knew what it wanted. It was sometimes suggested that political motives and trade balance were sometimes behind their demands. I saw no evidence of this. I believe that their requirements were not always properly understood and as a result were not met as simply and economically as they might have been.

The cost to the meat industry of this upheaval was enormous. Very large amounts of money were spent on what was euphemistically termed 'hygiene requirements'. These were being determined by American and New Zealand vets, but it always surprised me that within their respective departments the industry employed few if any professional veterinary advisors. Because of this dearth of professional advice the industry had no technical capacity to question or suggest alternatives. Even the Meat Industry Research Institute, a farmer funded organisation, did not have a vet on its staff.

The industry seemed to me to have enormous capacity to compound and complicate. After all, at the end of the day the objective was to provide clean, unadulterated meat, accurately labelled to the consumer. If this had been kept in mind more often, integrity maximised and suspicions minimised, then much time, money and effort could have been saved.

In many ways the New Zealand Department of Agriculture became an extension of its United States equivalent and was disposed to emulate rather than innovate.

Few meat plants were ever banned for long and the flow of hamburger meat across the Pacific continued in increasing volume to the country's considerable economic advantage. Unlike some other countries where export meat labelled beef was found on arrival in the U.S. to be of equine or marsupial origin, the New Zealand product soon proved to have the lowest rejection rate world-wide for any meat entering America.

The same regulations, however irksome, protected New Zealand from competition with countries such as South America. If its vast beef production had been allowed access to the American market in other then canned form, it would undoubtedly have seriously depressed the price which New Zealand received. However, the presence of diseases such as foot and mouth invoked regulatory control by the Americans. They could not afford to have a disease like foot and mouth run riot in their own enormous flocks and herds.

The part-time work offered me at Moerewa was 30 shillings an hour plus mileage to and from home. With a young family to sustain and two already at expensive schools, here was an opportunity to underpin the practice I was negotiating to start and few thought would succeed. After a lot of thought, because like most of my colleagues I preferred working with the living rather than the dead, I applied and was assigned half of the five working days of each week. Moerewa was one of the country's largest freezing works and only ten miles down the road.

I had, however, other reasons for my new commitment. I had long felt that the Veterinary Surgeon should be a guardian of animal welfare and it was clear to me that a place with a very high throughput of livestock could perhaps offer opportunity for the uncaring and unkind with no voice to represent the silent majority. I am glad to be able to say that I did not find a great deal of conscious cruelty in plants with which I became involved, consistent with these being parlours of death. I am also able to say that from time to time I was able to encourage better conditions to make the last hours of the animals I loved more tenable. Sometimes I was active in trying to limit unconscious cruelty.

My other reason for acting as I did was the belief that the meat industry offered an outstanding opportunity for the veterinary profession to become involved in the most significant and wealthiest sector in the country. However, the clinically oriented profession often seemed to regard colleagues who were so involved as something like second class citizens who had betrayed their calling.

Early in January 1964 I entered the gates of A.F.F.Co. into an environment as novel as it was new. It was natural that I was regarded by the meat inspection staff then working there as something of an intruder. This new boss from the blue was received with a degree of understandable apprehension. They need have had no fear. The new paper boss, while he may have known a bit about animals in the paddock, was quite at sea when it came to converting them to legs of lamb or sirloin steaks to grace the tables of the world.

A new vocabulary needed to be learned. On my second day as I passed a senior inspector on the stairs, he casually mumbled 'two o' clock' and passed on. 'What,' I thought 'could that mean?'

I later discovered that this piece of useful information was the forecast of the time work for the day would cease — apparently by far the most significant event to come.

Although I did not hear any new swear words here, their use was more sophisticated, with a variation in modulation and a fluency I had not before met. I once confounded a foreman, who was ranting on about something he couldn't or wouldn't do and which in any case I did not understand, by telling him that I only spoke English.

At this stage it was made clear to me that I was being paid for a presence to meet an American requirement. I was not really expected to do anything, although perhaps for appearance's sake I had been provided with a knife, a steel and a pouch. Half-a-dozen white coats completed my outfit.

One of the early problems was that although I was officially the meat inspector's boss I could not hope to match their expertise when it came to knife work. They sliced mostly invisible lymphatic nodes with a speed and accuracy that astonished me and which I could never match. I had been in this situation before in my army days. I was sometimes called upon to examine farriers although my expertise in shoeing a horse was at a very low level. It is not always necessary to be able to do something to judge whether or not it has been done well. This piece of philosophy I found difficult to impart to my new charges, who were at best helpful and at worst tolerant.

One perhaps surprising influence which limited my early progress in this field was noise, an excess of which I had never appreciated. There was an incessant cacophony of steel on concrete, cog on cog, the hiss of compressed air coupled with the crash of hooves and the splash of hearts and other things as they sped down chutes to nether regions for further attention. It was an assault on ears used to the more gentle murmurs of home and countryside. Longer standing employees seemed to have adjusted their auditory apparatus in such a way as to be able to communicate with each other despite the commotion all around.

There is always a story worth telling and this one involves my early days in the freezing works.

I had been called to conduct a pregnancy test on about half-a-dozen cows belonging to one of my more difficult clients. As I soaped my arm as a prelude to the necessary rectal palpation I asked my client if he had provided himself with a notebook to record the details for possible future reference.

'No need for all that,' said the farmer brusquely. 'I know all these cows by name and when you milk them twice a day like me you don't need to write things in books.'

'So be it,' I thought.

I determined that four of the cows were pregnant and two not so. My client, none too happy with my verdict, remarked that the job didn't look all that difficult and perhaps I could teach him sometime. I said that perhaps I could.

About two weeks later I was crossing to the village post office when I was hailed by a familiar voice.

'Hey,' said the voice. 'You know these cows you tested a while back?'

I said that I recollected the visit.

'Well,' said my client, 'one you said was empty was in calf'

'How,' I queried, ' do you know that?'

'There was a joker round selling brushes at the weekend — he reckoned he was a meat doctor at the works so I asked him to check up on these two cows I sent in — just to make sure like. Anyhow, he rang last night and said one was empty but one was in calf.'

Comment in such circumstances would have contributed little and I made none. The next day at the works I made it my business to find out which meat inspector was involved in the weekend brush trade and conveyed my displeasure concerning the information he had divulged.

The matter however did not rest there, for within a few days my client visited the surgery to pick up some medicine for an ailing calf.

'That story about the cow not being in calf was crook,' said the farmer. 'I must have got the numbers mixed up and sent in the wrong cow!'

Again, no comment was needed or forthcoming.

The Rewards of the Sixties

It became my habit to carry out urgent clinical work before breakfast, or perhaps en route to the freezing works where I spent a few hours each day. My afternoons were spent tuberculin testing. In the busy season the testing programme was suspended and I had time for more clinical cases.

The farm was also undergoing a process of evolution and this engaged a fair proportion of my mental capacity if not physical presence. The fences were slowly being upgraded and a start made with the construction of a race through the middle of the farm to the cowshed. It was fast becoming clear that Highway 1 was no place for cows to be twice a day on the way to and from the cowshed. Many truckloads of what was locally known as rotten rock was needed for the race. This soft rock, crushed and graded by heavy machinery, soon settled to form a hard surface which the herd could traverse even in the wettest weather. Ditches on either side were needed to drain off surface water, while concrete pipes were installed below the new race to encourage water to flow underneath and so reach natural channels. Eventually these emptied into the nearby stream.

The hills at the back of the farm across the stream attracted my attention although I was at first at a loss as to where to begin. In some places the slope was not too far off the vertical, and to the north was the pa. Its terraced fortifications were like the rest of the hill country, covered in gorse. I decided that if a track could be formed along this ridge it would act as a firebreak and a controlled burn-off of the gorse-covered slopes would be possible. I could then re-plant the area.

First I had to find a bulldozer operator who was skilled and perhaps foolhardy enough to negotiate the steep slopes into the gorse-shrouded territory. I was also a bit concerned about Maori sensitivities over the pa, but discreet enquiry revealed that it had no special standing as a place of reverence. In any case, the gorse was doing nothing for its aesthetic appeal, and I reasoned that the removal of this obnoxious weed might restore something of its former glory.

I discovered an industrious bulldozer operator on a farm where I was tuberculin testing and he promised to have a look. The problems which I had considered major seemed minor to this intrepid fellow. It did not take him long to carve quite a wide track from south-west to north-east along our northern boundary, proceeding along one of the steps of the pa and avoiding damage. Before he left he carted up a few hundred heavy concrete posts and strategically placed them where I hoped to erect a fence.

The idea was to burn off in three separate blocks although I was apprehensive about setting light to the gorse. It was of the 'old man' variety and would surely burn with intensity. I was not sure where any fire I started might end up if it jumped our firebreak, for it would have around 800 acres to work on. With a number of farms and buildings close by. I did not want to be held responsible for their incineration. I need not have worried for the matter was soon to be taken out of my hands. One hot summer while I was away in Wellington some other land developer or careless picnicker started a fire three or four miles away near Waimate North. Fanned by an easterly breeze the inferno spread with increasing venom over our property, ignoring the firebreaks. It was checked only when it reached the bank of our stream and the grassed paddocks of our farm provided less fuel on which the conflagration could feed. This was both good and bad news. It was good because it was an excellent burn-off in the hottest days of summer when I would not myself have dared to apply a match to the tinder dry brush. The bad news was that an orderly development was now history and pressure for seeding and fencing became urgent. If the dormant seeds of gorse were allowed to sprout again, within a short time the hills would again be covered by this aggressive legume.

So seed was spread, the new boundary fence erected, the Fletcher aircraft spread fans of fertiliser on the hungry hills and the bank balance retreated in confusion. The hills above Taiamai overlooking much of that ancient central basin were again about to become productive, most likely with the blessing of the souls of those long departed who lived, cultivated, fought and prospered in and around the pa.

The airstrip from which the fertiliser was spread only required the partial removal of one obstructing fence to make it functional and allow the heavily loaded aircraft to take off. The strip sloped downhill from the house and ran very close and parallel to Highway 1. This was really very convenient as the trucks of fertiliser and the mechanical loader which were needed to place the stuff in the aircraft, could operate within a few yards of the road gate. Passing traffic often watched the operation, and the local schoolmaster, perhaps anxious to escape the more mundane routine of the classroom, sometimes took his pupils to observe what was then a fairly new development in the world of agriculture. Distribution of fertiliser was thus quickly and efficiently achieved. But not always. One day the plane after dropping its load, skimmed low over the house and waggled its wings. A weight dropped from the pilot's seat accurately found its target on the front lawn.

'Lost a wheel. Gone to Kaitaia to land. Tell Reg.' said the note wrapped round the dropped spanner.

The pilot again waggled his wings and set off for Kaitaia where there were superior emergency services. I later found the missing wheel beside a rocky outcrop halfway down the airstrip but well to the left. Reg, the plane's owner, came over from Kaikohe to pick up the missing wheel, expressing wonderment as to why the pilot had been so far off-course. I later found out that the aircraft had made a successful landing on one wheel on the grass at Kaitaia airport.

On another occasion the hopper jammed and a near full load of fertiliser was inadvertently dropped on the roof of a house in the village. This caused some consternation as the rainwater off the roof was the only source of domestic supply, and now it was contaminated. I believe the owner of the house and the top-dressing company negotiated a settlement, although what it was I never found out.

My German sharemilker finally decided that cows were not for him and I was once again placed in the difficult situation of finding suitable labour. I had come to know a Dutchman named John Dolfing who had recently taken up a sharemilking contract at *Northlands* at Waimate North with some 600 acres, half in grass. This farm was the one which John Duncan had discussed with me in San Francisco. Dolfing told me that he had a friend called Marinus Traas, not long arrived from Holland and at that time working on a small dairy farm near Palmerston North. This worker was anxious to expand his horizons and prospects and correspondence was followed with an interview. The happy result was that Rinus, as we were to call him, and his newly acquired wife Gae, were soon installed in our cottage. So began an amicable and productive association of some 12 years. It would be fair to say that without the dedication and particularly the stability which Rinus provided, I would not later have had the confidence to project our enterprise into the rewarding but exacting fields of town milk production and stud cattle breeding, which contributed so much to eventual success.

With a new milker installed for the 1962 season, things were looking fairly stable. Although important policy decisions were soon to be taken I felt able to accede to John Duncan's request and take over the supervision of *Northlands*. I thus became more involved with the affairs of that place, and especially with John Dolfing.

Northlands had once been something of a showpiece but had slipped badly, most likely as a result of indifferent management. The volcanic land was of high quality, but fencing was primitive and stock quality poor. Dolfing told me that when he took over the management he had to retrieve a number of cows gone bush in the scrub, and on one occasion had to take refuge on the roof of the cowshed to escape the attentions of an irate bovine, resentful at being reintroduced to the boring routine of commercial dairying.

I do not believe that John Duncan was aware of the tiger he had by the tail, in an economic sense. All the cows were destined for the American hamburger market as soon as they could be replaced by more peaceful and productive substitutes. Fences needed to be replaced and fertiliser had to be applied to pastures which urgently needed rejuvenating.

The big, old kauri house had seen better days, although it was basically of sound construction. It was one of the earlier homes in a district famed for its historic buildings, and must have been all of a century old. There was little cash available for home improvement but the indomitable Dolfing and his chainsaw soon converted two rooms into one to better suit the needs of his family. His possessions included a large organ which he operated proficiently and played occasionally to entertain visitors like myself.

Feeling his farm was understocked, John Duncan — unknown to Dolfing or myself — purchased about 40 head of in-calf Poll Angus cows in the Wairarapa and despatched them to *Northlands*. Angus cows look at things in a different way from dairy stock, and after some days in trucks a few wires across their path weren't going to stop them. The wide open spaces of the north had a lot of appeal. Most of the new beef herd quickly disappeared into the bush and scrub which covered around 300 acres at the back of the farm, pursued vigorously by John Dolfing Junior on horseback. Efforts to recover the erring stock or 'bullocks', as Dolfing inaccurately called them, were not immediately successful. But as winter closed in a few bales of hay scattered at random at the edge of the scrub gradually tempted them out of their refuge and contact was fortunately re-established before their calves were born.

John Duncan was never a satisfied owner, even if the production was raised from 16,000 lbs to 36,000 lbs of butterfat in a couple of years. Looking at figures behind his desk in Wellington led him to the conclusion that farming in the north was not quite as profitable as he had hoped. He sometimes came up and toured the property on the tractor's tray. When he saw the green pastures and breathed the country air I think he felt better, showing it by exuding old-world charm to all around.

Towards the end of the decade John decided to sell the property to realise a profit. By coincidence John Dolfing eventually bought the first old house we had owned and he lives there to this day. His optimism, industry, sense of humour, and use of English which might have given Mrs Malaprop a few ideas, made him a good neighbour to a few fortunates and a friend to many more. From time to time we still visit John and his good wife, killing as it were, two birds with the one stone. Old acquaintance extends to the house as well as its owner.

I was slowly becoming convinced that the Friesian breed might have a better future in New Zealand than the long-established Jersey. It looked as if solids might be more the basis for calculating payment than the less desirable butter fat. Although it was illogical to base decision-making on experience with one animal, our first Friesian, Bonny Choice, was a top producer and impressed me greatly. Among my clients were Steadman Brothers who farmed difficult country a few miles back from Moerewa. Their long-established Friesian stud *Ellerlea* produced well, despite the poor hills and wet flats which they farmed. One famous daughter, Ellerlea Wakalona Petal, in the hands of Alan Billington of Whangarei, was New Zealand's top cow of the year on one occasion.

Claud Steadman was of great assistance to us in our early years for we had decided to expand our interest in Friesian cattle and had joined the Breed Society. I always attended the annual sales at Steadmans' and made such purchases as appealed and we could afford. Claud also made one of his better bulls available to us at no charge, and so the stud was soon on its way.

But every stud had to have a name. Our land was strewn with stone and rocky outcrop, some stacked like monumental cairns in a country far away. There was also a backdrop of hills, so the name *Cairnhill* almost suggested itself. It also happened to be the name of a district in my Scottish hometown. To this day *Cairnhill* is being successfully farmed, although in a different part of the country and under different ownership.

The colour of the grazing herd, in line with our policy, was changing from Jersey grey or gold to black and white which stood out against the green pastures. When the first pedigree calves arrived they had to be identified by photographing their right side on which the white patches, never the same, stood out like the maps of some unknown land.

An important part of keeping in touch with farming operations was by recording the production of each cow. This took place each month when the tester employed by the local herd improvement association called and stayed the night. In the early times the testers travelled between farms on a horse-drawn cart. This mode of transport cost little and travelled fast enough to make the usually short journeys between farms practical, although it exposed the passenger to the vagaries of the weather. As the testers, some of whom were female, had to spend each night in a different place, their reception and conditions of board were much varied and some quite startling tales were indeed told. By coincidence, the testers could become quite intimately involved in family affairs like weddings, christenings and even funerals. One girl told me that during her stay in one place a burglar unwisely attempted to ply his trade in the farmhouse, only to be discovered by an irate farmer who discharged both barrels of his shotgun in his direction. The spreading shot missed the fleeing intruder, but not by much.

The testing operation itself consisted of measuring the volume of milk produced by each cow — morning and evening. A simple calculation revealed the amount of butterfat each cow had produced and if this was multiplied by the number of days in the month the all-important monthly production was revealed. At the end of the lactation, the still more important annual figure could be calculated. Carting heavy buckets of milk from cowshed to milk room, and then tipping the contents into the vat was heavy work, especially for a young woman, but most seemed to manage.

Another important decision soon had to be made. Town milk was needed for the district's many schools and townships, the burgeoning tourist industry, and even for sheep farmers. The latter were becoming less inclined to milk a troublesome house cow each day. The farmers also had to contend with the milk provider's veterinary problems and, in any case, the cow was dry for quite a part of the year. Half-a-dozen or so town milk producers supplied the milk treatment station in Kaikohe. The station pasteurised and bottled the milk and then distributed it to the various milk vendors of the district.

Jack Byers, the farmer and race commentator whom I had known for a number of years, was chairman of the local town milk suppliers and was anxious for us to fill a vacancy in the local town milk supply. Perhaps more so than some of his fellow farmers, he had a confidence in our ability to deliver the goods, and we were also very centrally located.

I was not too enthusiastic at accepting a binding contract because I was virtually an absentee owner dependent on others to milk the cows. Apart from the better returns which naturally appealed to my Scottish streak, there were one or two points in favour. First of all, the farm was well suited for milking through the wet and often muddy winters because it was mostly on easy-draining volcanic soil. I had also been anxious for some time to move away from pigs, despite it being quite profitable. Pigs required heavy labour input with daily feeding, cleaning, supervision and separation of cream. True, the piggery had been improved with a couple of farrowing pens added but these could be adapted to house calves, whose numbers I expected to increase as the number of stud cows in the herd grew.

After a long and very frank discussion with my manager, Rinus, and some careful budgeting, I decided to go ahead. I was granted a daily quota of 80 gallons, which wasn't a lot but quite enough. The herd had to be turned around with more than half the cows made to calve from late January through

April to ensure the quota was maintained over the winter months. The cowshed also had to be upgraded to meet town milk standards, and a milk vat, cooler and other equipment purchased.

An early problem was to provide a track for the large milk tanker to gain access to the cowshed. There was no great difficulty for the first 200 yards or so from the road, but in the vicinity of the cowshed a rocky outcrop had to be bulldozed away to provide a circular track for the tanker to turn. This was eventually accomplished, although some pretty large boulders needed to be pushed aside and the track was really always a bit on the steep side. An inexperienced driver sometimes failed to persuade his heavily-laden tanker to leave, without the extra horsepower provided by the farm tractor hitched on ahead.

I was under pressure from various advisors to install a more modern milking machine but this I resisted. I had noted that when travelling round the district that a number of herringbone milking sheds were being built. These often incorporated a new and improved performance milking machine which operated at high vacuum pressure. This enabled one man to quickly milk quite a large number of cows. I formed the opinion though that when this happened, the cups were left on the cows too long and after all the milk in their udders had been removed. This resulted in the powerful machine-generated vacuum causing bruising to the teat orifice. Specks of blood could sometimes be detected, an ideal medium for bacteria causing mastitis to multiply. The proverb of swings and roundabouts applied. Time saved in milking was often more than offset by treating mastitis-afflicted cows.

Most of the carpentry in the cowshed was carried out by Colin Smith who also owned a small farm not far away. Some time before Colin had built a substantial double car-port for us at the house without apparently having obtained the necessary building permit from the county council. A good location has its disadvantages, for Colin's indiscretion was noted by the building inspector who one day strode down our drive with battle in his eye, as I was discussing progress with my builder.

'Gentlemen, gentlemen what have we here?' queried the bespectacled and angry inspector, surveying the near-completed edifice.

I didn't have the right answer so I left it to Colin, who must have been successful in pacifying the inspector for he applied no penalty. When I later passed through the new car-port Colin made no comment apart from mumbling indecipherables under his breath.

In my dairy farm philosophy I was influenced by McMeekan and his book *Grass to Milk* which had appeared about the same time as we went farming. However, town milk was a bit more complicated and as production had to be achieved under all weather conditions it became clear to me that because grass could not always be guaranteed other ways of feeding stock had to be found. The New Zealand farmer was, and still is, very much wedded to his grass. Whenever it disappeared he was left in crisis, promptly appealing to a usually benevolent government for assistance. This was often in the form of a subsidy covering the importation of hay or temporarily shifting stock to another part of the country where the grass still grew. All this was fine, but it didn't help the town dweller who liked to enjoy milk in his tea or even the odd milkshake, or the town milk supplier who was under contract.

My system of management was based on the incomparable McMeekan when the grass grew, but when it didn't I had to look elsewhere. I found renewed knowledge and indeed comfort in one of my old text books with the rather ponderous title of *Animal Nutrition and Veterinary Dietetics*. This book quoted older times in Britain in which cows, to be close to the urban market for their milk, were actually housed in the city. All their sustenance, such as hay and roots, was delivered to them. There was no grass for such cows, although according to my book they still produced close on four gallons each day; so why panic here?

The problem looked to be organisational, needing to be founded on planning and purchase. The planning was to ensure that maximum reserves were built up from the farm in time of plenty and to be prepared to put our money where our mouth was; if we wanted to sustain a high quota we were going to have to make substantial financial outlay buying extra hay and especially concentrate in the form of dairy meals which were not of particularly high quality or variety. In practice, it meant that in spring we harvested as much of the farm as was possible for silage. This was chiefly as an insurance against droughts. Buying hay or even meal was not always easy and availability was a continuing matter of concern.

Some grass-minded agriculturalists will no doubt dispute my technique on economic grounds, but I believe that under the town milk system it paid off. In conditions of severe drought, for instance, we did not have the cows expend energy by driving them to and from some distant paddock, brown and bare and with no nutritional value. Instead they were allowed to browse on a rocky slope by the cowshed where the stream flowed and shade was provided by the canopy of willows above. In such a place, it was possible to feed the ample ration of silage, supplemented at milking times by an appropriate allowance of meal dispensed through the hoppers in the cowshed. Our production hardly ever fell below four gallons a day for each cow. We could maintain our quota with seldom more than 50 or 60 cows going through the shed in times of stress; fewer to feed and milk and worry about, but enough to meet our contractual obligations just the same.

This heavy feeding/high yield per cow philosophy had another spin-off.

As a vet I was impressed with the fact that our herd appeared to have fewer serious veterinary problems than those which depended on grass alone. Bloat and grass staggers were largely absent, and milk fever and mastitis minimal.

As our performance improved so too did the quota allocated to us and as we were by now one of the larger producers, I was asked to stand for and was subsequently elected to the directorate of the Bay of Islands Cooperative Milk Producers. I enjoyed this new responsibility into which from time to time I introduced new perspectives. I occasionally represented the directorate at the annual conference of the national organisation and there met a number of long-established and affluent town milk producers who continued to defend their status and economic structure with vigour and determination. The industry was heavily subsidised by central government and was thus under continual pressure, resisted on the grounds that the burden of producing milk the year round on contract was an onerous responsibility which justified every penny received. This was most likely a fair claim, although to me it was never quite clear why a government subsidy was needed to prop a product which the public would have bought in any case.

By the mid-sixties the herd was perhaps half stud Friesian. I had also made a few excellent purchases locally from farmers like Jock Murray who sold us an outstanding artificially-bred matron, Puriri Glen Barbara. We started to spread our wings and travel to sales further afield hoping to add new talent to our enterprise. I remember buying twin heifers at the Sunnybrae sale near Auckland Airport. One calved before she could be sent north and studmaster Archie Montgomery was reluctant to send a newly born calf such a long way by truck. He suggested we pick up a replacement at a later convenient time. This we did, and I well remember collecting a nearly all black calf we called Sunnybrae who proved to be one of the most pleasant members of the herd. Sunnybrae travelled back to Ohaeawai in the boot of the Holden with frequent stops to make sure our cherished acquisition was still able to breathe. By now the roads were better and I had replaced my last Landrover with a car.

Another way we improved the herd was by the use of artificial breeding and nominating the bulls we felt would best improve our herd's prospects. The insemination was done by technicians employed by the local herd improvement association which also ran the herd testing scheme we were already patronising. The technician, sometimes called the 'bull in the bowler hat' was notified early each day if any of the cows were in receptive mood. He soon arrived with a supply of semen stored in a flask of liquid nitrogen and initiated a new life to make its earthly impact some nine months later. In the early days the bulls selected for use were chosen on a basis of the production alone of their ancestry with little thought given to conformation.

This shortcoming was later corrected but meantime it had to be watched. It was not good business to breed a cow genetically capable of extraordinarily high production if her udder dragged so close to the ground that it was impossible to apply the cups of the milking machine to recover the promised milky bonanza. While the purist was often chided because he might place looks, temperament and conformation before production all aspects were needed and the first three often complemented the fourth.

By 1968 the herd was predominantly stud Friesian and I mustered sufficient confidence to arrange for a sale of surplus stock. Alongside the race we had built a corrugated iron pavilion which doubled as extra storage space for hay, which on sale day we arranged in tiers to provide seating for the buyers and usually greater number of spectators. On the opposite side of the race the farm trailer, still attached to the tractor, was parked to act as a rostrum for the auctioneers. A tarpaulin was draped and secured over a galvanised frame to keep out any rain. This arrangement kept out most of the rain, but not all wind which in May could be quite chilly. Stock agents, used to a more protected environment, were not all that complimentary.

It was with bated breath that we awaited the arrival of the much hoped for buyers. As the scheduled start time approached it seemed that only ourselves and some stock agents, enjoying the morning tea provided, might prove to be the only ones around. However, a couple of full cars driven by stock agents from the south arrived, and a few other unpredictable figures wearing gum boots, oilskins and other protective clothing trudged in from the road. We ended up starting 20 minutes late to a reasonably full bench. The stock was driven up the race and held between two gates for the attention of the buyers. I too was in this erstwhile sale ring armed with a light stick ostensibly to gently move the offering of the moment to and fro while explaining its virtues to the buyers assembled.

One or two of the offering did not appreciate this new type of exposure and one heifer in particular eyed me with disfavour. She stopped opposite, pawed the ground, snorted and nodded her head as angry cows do, and looked as if she would attack at any moment. I was sorely tempted to scale the gate but a vendor who flees from his offering is no advertisement at all. I stood my ground very still and whispered what I hoped were soothing words to a bovine. My heifer paused, considered the situation and turned her attention to the noisy and loquacious auctioneer who, fortunately for him, was out of reach. He later congratulated me on my fortitude. Another of the offering did not stop to be sold at all but skilfully leapt the enclosing gate and another fence before disappearing over the horizon, surprisingly pursued by several bids from those assembled. Temperament apparently, wasn't everything!

Obviously our first sale was not an unqualified success and maybe a bit premature. Prices were on the low side but it was a start, and it gave us experience to build on. It soon became an annual event held in the May school holidays. We eventually combined forces with three other local breeders and the expanded offering encouraged a greater attendance. There was, like everything else worthwhile, a considerable amount of preparatory work

needed, such as the preparation of the catalogues which recorded the past performance of the ancestors of the stock on offer. Heifers offered as in calf had to be examined by the resident vet to make sure that this was in fact the case. Substantial cooking and baking was needed to feed the hungry buyers and spectators, and even a few dozen beers had to be tucked away for the hoped for after-sale celebration. Trucks, sometimes bound for distant parts, operated far into the night taking the stock to their new homes. Always a red letter day for us, the sale days are among the happiest of my memories.

Another pleasing activity which emerged as our stock improved was the opportunity to exhibit some at the local agricultural shows, chiefly at Kaikohe and Waimate North. For us these shows were no one day affair, but meant weeks of grooming and leading before the day of judgement. On the day, the final touches needed to be applied before the truck arrived to take the sometimes reluctant competitors to show. Our stock did not always behave themselves as well as they might have but, nonetheless, over the years a good number of blue and red and yellow prize ribbons adorned bedroom walls. It was very much a family effort for all contributed, and thus it was all the more pleasurable.

The Breezes of Change

As the sixties approached its autumn, the breezes of change started to make themselves felt like the wood smoke of some fire, uncertain in its direction but bound to go somewhere.

The years of calving cows and my other duties, often carried out in wet and windy places, had started to take their toll on me. An incipient, but luckily painless arthritis of my fingers had started to develop. I sadly came to the conclusion that my days in practice would have to end a bit earlier than I had supposed. Strength of hand and sureness of touch are necessary attributes for the vet in the field.

The situation in New Zealand was a bit different than in the older countries such as Britain where a long-established veterinary practice developed an intrinsic value based on the goodwill it had generated. Senior partners holding the majority shareholding often retained this while acting as a consultant to their more youthful colleagues. This provided a depth of experience to patient and client while allowing the senior to retain a less demanding, but welcome interest. But in my day Jack was as good as his master and the boss was expected to foot it with the rest. I was sorry to leave my clients, some of whom may well have felt that I was abandoning them for material gain, although the reason was far from that. I had some regrets that the system of free enterprise I had generated was about to revert to the club, for although I had advertised my intentions and promised assistance to establish, there was surprisingly no interest.

The Meat Division had been keen for me to accept an offer of veterinary supervision at Moerewa freezing works on a full-time basis. This sort of work caused a degree of aggravation in a number of ways but digital arthritis was not one of them. The other advantage was that the workplace was near the farm which by now had become my consuming interest. I decided to accept the offer but before I donned the protective, if sometimes frustrating, mantle of the public servant I made one more trip to Scotland.

I decided this time that I should take advantage of my necessary journey to visit places I had not been before. I therefore booked an Air India flight across Australia's desolate interior to Perth. After a night there, Qantas took me across the Indian Ocean to the green plantations of Mauritius and thence on to Johannesburg high on the veldt of South Africa. I stayed five days in South Africa and to me it looked rich and prosperous. There was no sign of poverty that I could detect, but it was a difficult place to feel welcome with the black inhabitants passing with apparently unseeing eyes, acknowledging no recognition of their white fellow pedestrian.

I journeyed to Pretoria across a golden brown veldt dotted with the massive mole hills of the gold workings. In some ways it reminded me of Curacao in the Caribbean for in both places the Dutch had a dominating influence. A look at Soweto was from a distance, for my taxi driver thought it wise not to go too close. It was then northwards in a VC10 of B.O.A.C., above nearly the entire length of Africa, across the Mediterranean with the lights of Rome to starboard, and landing at Heathrow at night. There was one stop in this journey; the plane swung in low over Lake Victoria to land at Entebbe. The passengers were not permitted to disembark as fresh fuel was pumped aboard, and there was little incentive to do so. Armed soldiers, dressed in camouflage clothing matching a few DC-3 aircraft parked nearby, appeared anything but friendly.

My father, now a sprightly 85-year-old, was still active although very much alone, for his sisters had all departed for a higher destiny. His isolation did not seem to cause him great concern though for he had long been a loner as well as a survivor.

I clearly had to make some arrangements about *Wallcroft*, the family home and what was in it, including the sole occupant. I started by visiting my old school, Glasgow High, where the rector put me in touch with James B. Highgate. He was a well-known lawyer practising in the city and he had been a contemporary of mine at school before the war. It so happened that Jimmy Highgate was also active in the Presbyterian Church and was acquainted with Tom Jardine Johnstone, who on our first visit to Scotland had christened our son. The minister, with whom I still correspond, was also well known to my father who regarded him with considerable respect — unusual for one who, for the most part, steered clear of men of the cloth.

A friend of my late Aunt Lizzie, a Miss Lindsay Gibson, had transferred her affinity for my aunt to her brother. I was therefore most fortunate to be able to establish a caring triumvirate, able and willing to assist my father if he ever needed help and could ever bring himself to accept it.

I arranged for most of the heavy furniture to be sold and most of what was transportable to be sent to New Zealand. This was a very difficult decision for me but I could see that unless I took the initiative, the family silver would most likely just evaporate. I also had to become involved physically, for stored in the cellar below the house were all sorts of relics retrieved from the family grocery business when it came time to close the door for the last time. Cases of canned food, counters and drawers, bacon slicers and display cabinets were there in profusion. These mementoes of another time were now mere debris so I hired a 'skip' from the borough council to take it away. I was not sorry to see the suspended skip disappear down Finlaystone Street heading for parts unknown.

I hired a chauffeur-driven Daimler for a week, and with my father and sometimes Miss Gibson as passengers, we visited places we had known long ago and which had nostalgic memories; perhaps more so for my father, for I think he had visited the same places with my mother before my time. From Edinburgh on the Forth to Glasgow on the Clyde and its glorious Firth beyond, we journeyed in style. We drove from Stirling, the gateway to the Highlands and whose name we bore, to Peebles and the soft, tranquil beauty of the Border country where walls and farmhouses of stone gave an impression of permanence not often sensed in other places. It was a journey down memory lane and the valley of time.

Before I left I gave my lawyer full power-of-attorney. My father clearly wanted to bide where he was and this time, perhaps being older and wiser, I could more easily see his point of view. He survived three more years and was well cared for in his last few months until age finally won the day. *Wallcroft* was sold and although we have since visited the old place it no longer seems quite the same as it was in the golden years of long ago.

I returned to New Zealand via Hong Kong where I spent a hectic five days under the tutelage of a Chinese guide who shifted me with alacrity from the Tiger Balm Gardens to the frontier with China and a lot of other places in-between. His main ambition though seemed to be to escape the milling masses of his homeland and make a new life in uncluttered New Zealand of which he had heard glowing reports. I hope he realised his dream for he was a likeable chap.

An unscheduled stop in the middle of the night at Manila gave me the chance to pick up a few exotic presents before returning exhausted but content to the place I knew best.

One day early in 1970 I had a telephone call from the president of the New Zealand Veterinary Association, the national organisation which represented all vets practising within the country. Association president Reg Trounson wanted to know if I would be prepared to serve on the council. After a bit of thought I agreed to serve, although the monthly meetings held in

Hamilton meant a long drive, leaving early Saturday and arriving home late Sunday.

I was surprised at the breadth and complexity of the issues we dealt with and sometimes wondered if councillors like myself had the background to make useful contributions. Disciplinary problems, professional fees, doping, tuberculosis, hydatids, animal remedies and plenty more involved the Association. I felt the meetings interesting, but exhausting and they often left me unfulfilled.

I also think that I failed in what was meant to be my main function which was to act as a liaison between my Northland branch and the parent body. I was still a member of the National Hydatids Council and of course my daily bread and butter came from my work at the Moerewa works. When I came up for re-election at the annual conference in Wellington in 1971 I was defeated by Peter Malone, now mayor of Nelson. The reason, I believe, was perhaps a lack of support from my home base and, perhaps more importantly a member of the Meat Division was not seen as a particularly suitable representative for the clinically oriented and more numerous sector which earned its living by restoring life and not presiding over its demise. Fair enough too, I guess.

The farm had by now about reached about its peak of efficiency. In the 1971-72 season 75 cows had averaged 436 lbs milk fat and topped the testing group. The town milk quota had risen to 175 gallons each day and would rise another twenty. The annual sales were also attracting increasing attention. I had been joined by two of my old clients, Jim Halliday and Arthur White, and we were collectively able to submit around 50 head for sales. The name *Cairnhill* began to have increasing significance in the round of dairy sales held each winter around May.

To this day I still ask myself why it was with all this apparent achievement and the hard work done, we decided to put *Cairnhill* on the market. I suppose that the catalyst was when my long-standing manager Rinus announced he wanted a change and had purchased a horticultural property at Kerikeri. This I could understand for milking cows, especially someone else's day by day and year-in year-out, must have limited fascination for most. Of course, a replacement could have been found but of what standard?

Having reached the limit of its potential the farm now required fairly fine tuning to keep it right. It was efficient, highly commercial but not relaxing. I wanted a more direct participation for myself in the farm by driving a tractor more often, watching my animals graze the grass of summer, and observing the content and acknowledgement in the eyes of stock enjoying their hay in winter. I suppose I wanted to be alone more often where perhaps a stream tumbled into a silent pool; where tuis chorused and the plaintive cry of the morepork echoed in the night.The mathematics appeared right for a town milk farm commanded a premium above others. Although we set a fairly high price and there was virtually only one buyer interested, it was enough. We decided to let our head rule our heart and find a new place in the sun, which we eventually did. That is another story for another time, as it evolved some distance from the hills above Taiamai. I had however, graduated a second time — I felt I was a farmer at last.

Fellow Mortals

'I'm truly sorry man's dominion
Has broken nature's social union,
And justifies that ill opinion
Which makes thee startle,
At me, thy poor earth born companion
and fellow mortal.'

So wrote Robert Burns in 1785 when his plough accidentally destroyed the nest of a field mouse and sent its occupant scurrying in confusion over the rough stubble.

Do such sentiments still prevail over two centuries later? I think that they most likely do, but the picture is by no means clear cut.

I am often asked questions by interviewers on radio and by journalists, as well as by personal acquaintances, about the welfare of animals. Cases of gross cruelty to animals often feature in media outlets and these horrific acts rightly attract the disgust of most. The heavy hand of the justiciary dispenses severe, if sometimes still inadequate penalties to the perpetrators. Children sometimes give vent to their frustrations on their own or other pets, although such acts even if detected, are for obvious reasons not always publicised.

Dreadful as such individual acts of cruelty are, the number of cases in proportion to the animal population as a whole is most likely not high. The question needs to be asked whether cruelty should be measured by individual spectacular and horrifying acts perpetrated by a few or maybe by its less dramatic, but equally intense involvement of many. In the handling of animals I believe that familiarity does indeed sometimes induce contempt. In freezing works I detected few cases of deliberate cruelty, even if the odd employee did from time to time lose his temper and vent his spite on the nearest living thing. However, other things happened which perhaps could have been avoided or circumstances improved. I think the animals were too often considered part of the plant instead of, as Burns put it, fellow mortals.

I would have thought when technology was able to put a man on the moon, and shift a heart or maybe a kidney from a dead donor to an anxious but eager recipient, more sophisticated means might have been designed than the club and knife to end the time in this world for those who man needed for his sustenance or business. In the hands of experts such primitive tools were effective most of the time, although a very small percentage failure rate in 100,000 head a day is enough to cause significant suffering. I also wondered about the aesthetic aspect and whether it was appropriate to ask people to perform such tasks. I must say that those who did appeared to show no inhibition concerning their bloody and grisly work. Technology did intervene in the end and the electrical stunning of sheep at least became the norm.

Today things are better, if still some way to go, but I wondered why it took so long. The executioners were conditioned to it; management, I think, preferred a blind eye to a sympathetic ear so research in this important field lagged behind that directed at more profitable returns. It is not to this country's credit that the thrust for improvement in the end came from some of our overseas customers rather than from within.

There were other more blatant assaults on animal welfare. One which could easily have been stopped was the damage and suffering caused by bovine horns. Cattle have horns devised by nature to keep predators at bay and perhaps defend their young. In open spaces these sometimes long and sharp appendages do little harm but when cattle are yarded or trucked, stock unused to the close proximity of their peers often become aggressive. They use their horns as punishing weapons.

I recall one case in which around 30 head of horned cattle were despatched from Kaitaia to a freezing works in Auckland for slaughter because that was where the best price could be obtained. Before the halfway point was reached half the load had succumbed to the attack of their mates. The owner, chastened by his losses, sent the next consignment to a plant nearer home. But in this first case, although there were no fatalities, the bloodied and bruised meat surrounding holes where horns had penetrated was a disturbing sight.

Horn growth can be fairly easily prevented by chemical or electrical treatment of the new horn buds soon after birth, and horns may be removed later although an anaesthetic is sometimes required. It would have been easy enough to legislate to prohibit horned stock being accepted at freezing works. It would have been easy for management or truck firms to refuse to handle such stock. I guess it would have been reasonable to allow a period of grace to allow the adult horned stock to be filtered out of the system. In the end nothing effective happened at all, each suggesting the other should bite the bullet, claiming loss of business or maybe votes as an excuse. The debate and the carnage continued.

Another face of animal welfare surfaced when E.E.C. vets wanted stock in freezing works to be housed in covered yards to protect them from heat and cold.

'No way,' said farmers, management and many others. 'Our stock spend their life in the open so why do they have to be covered when they reach the works?'

The sense of outrage was considerable.

The concrete flooring of a pen can become very hot in the summer, so hot that the human hand cannot bear it. Perhaps bovine feet are a lot tougher? I have an open mind on this one although I am sure that covered yards made the work of those attending the stock a lot more pleasant. As for the stock at home on the farm — maybe it should have had some shade too!

Many city dwellers, perhaps fulfilling a long latent need, feel the desire for the companionship of some living thing like a dog or cat or bird or fish. Primitive man often used dogs to assist him in his hunting and this is reflected in the use of specially bred dogs to pursue a quarry. Sometimes they are used to frighten a concealed bird into flight and then, if the shot of the human master is accurate, retrieve the trophy from where it fell. Nowadays, a deteriorating social structure has led people to own a dog with the perceived purpose of discouraging would-be robbers or assailants.

The activities I have mentioned leave scope for what I term 'unconscious cruelty' where the animal is subject to varying degrees of cruelty but it is not perceived by the owner as such. Many large dogs are retained as pets but have to spend much of their life shut in a small flat while their owners work. The so-called sporting dog enjoys the wide open spaces for perhaps a few months of the year but the rest of the time has nowhere to go. He is confined in some pen or kennel where boredom may lead to his noisy expression of objection so causing a crisis in human relationship.

It is unfortunate that many city dwellers do not choose a breed which best suits their purpose. Large aggressive breeds have become increasingly popular, ostensibly for guard purposes but more often I think to reflect the machismo of their owners. A small fox terrier type would eat a lot less, and bark just as loudly if an intruder threatened. Large dogs need a few miles of exercise each day to keep them healthy and they also need constant and complete control lest they vent their natural aggression on some innocent victim. There is a wide range of small pet dogs which will suit the need of most, but even then, a pet should only be acquired if adequate and sustained attention can be given. A cat may be a better solution as on the whole they are easier to manage, eat less and some, like the Siamese and Burmese, have an unusual affinity for human company.

It is one thing to use an animal for sport. It is quite another to make it a target for it.

Bull fighting, still attracting many spectators in some parts of the world, is surely an appeal to a primitive blood lust which one would have thought many centuries of so-called civilisation would have moderated. An off-shoot in New Zealand is dog fighting, clandestinely arranged in some secret place but practised just the same. Pit bull terrier pups are advertised in the newspapers for up to $700; perhaps an indication of the purpose for which their use in intended?

Another sport for which I can find little enthusiasm is big game fishing. I believe the match between hunter and hunted is uneven. The angler, strapped in a custom-designed chair, has a considerable advantage over an adversary with a steel hook embedded in its mouth. The struggle is for many hours to the point of exhaustion. The game fish does not have the option of the hunter who can withdraw and call it a draw at any time. I especially abhor the practice of towing an exhausted fish backwards behind a powerful launch to hasten death by drowning and avoiding possible retaliation by the vanquished if hoisted on board. I am glad to see that fish caught nowadays are sometimes tagged and then released to fight another day — if they recover from the ordeal.

One practice, born of kindness, can cause much animal and indeed human anguish. When Christmas or birthday time comes around it sometimes happens that live animals are considered as being suitable gifts, particularly to children. The donor should be quite certain that such a gift is wanted and, more importantly, that the recipient has the resources and inclination to provide sustained love and care for the new charge. While in practice I had a number of blameless pets brought to me for euthanasia. Their owners had grown tired of their responsibility or could not fit them into their holiday or other social schedule. In other cases the unwanted were allowed to come and go as they pleased, creating a nuisance for others. By further breeding the problem compounded.

It is a comfort to know that large consignments of stock sent overseas nowadays are accompanied by a vet who supervises their welfare and reports on conditions of accommodation and method of management. Of course, life does not end at unloading and the hiatus in time between then and the moment of their slaughter should also be under scrutiny. Otherwise the exporting nation could become an inadvertent accessory to much suffering in a land in which it has little control but, as supplier of the stock, must surely have a continuing responsibility.

While being interviewed on radio I was asked what I considered was the most significant advance in veterinary science in recent times. My off-the-cuff answer was veterinary anaesthesia. The maxim that one has to be cruel to be kind found no greater expression than in the early days of veterinary practice. I suppose that human medicine must have had its parallels for I have a drawing of a screaming patient of the last century having his leg amputated by saw. The only anaesthetic visible is a discarded bottle which I suspect had held whisky rather than chloroform.

Certain procedures have always been necessary for reasons of commerce or commonsense. Lambs need to be docked and castrated for their own as well as commercial benefit. Cattle with long horns are a danger to themselves and others. The tails of cows perhaps need to be amputated to protect their attendants from discomfort or disease. Pets may need to be neutered to prevent a proliferation of unwanted progeny.

Some procedures, like the docking of some breeds of pups, are carried out to present a preconceived image of the breed involved. If the image changes so will the custom, and some very influential people and organisations seem that way inclined. In any event, if such an operation is performed at all it should be done under an anaesthetic.

The bovine has never been a good subject for general anaesthesia, largely because when they are recumbent, its commodious first stomach or rumen presses forward on the lungs and heart. It can also regurgitate contents into the throat from where inhalation can easily cause the bronchi to block or initiate a usually fatal pneumonia. Fortunately, the bovine is a good subject for local or regional anaesthesia. Many of the important sensory nerves are superficial and can be rendered insensitive by injecting a small amount of local anaesthetic over them. Operations like de-horning, removal of a foot claw, or even major ones like caesarian section, can be painlessly carried out using such a technique, perhaps supplemented by a tranquiliser to keep the patient placid.

The horse was always rather a better subject for anaesthesia than the cow, perhaps because its stomach was of less generous proportion. Chloroform administered through a sponge held in a canvas mask strapped over the head, or a solution of chloral hydrate administered via the jugular vein, produced a satisfactory result. Strangely enough, in older lands, there was sometimes considerable owner resistance to the use of anaesthetics. In the area of Scotland where I worked as a student the clientele thought little of a vet who needed to use an anaesthetic to castrate a colt. The opinion of the day was that such an operation needed only a sleight of hand and agility of foot on the part of the operator without any nonsense like anaesthesia. Nowadays, far more sophisticated anaesthetics are available, enabling even the most complex operations and procedures to be undertaken safely.

Anaesthesia has thus gradually been reducing the need to be cruel to be kind and although there is still some way to go — particularly where operative procedures are carried out by non professionals — I believe important advances have been made. All of which is gratifying for those of us who care for our friends on four legs, as well as appreciating their commercial and recreational significance to us.

My opinion was often sought as to whether the sustaining of an unhappy life in perhaps a long-owned and loved pet was justified or reasonable. I was always glad to give an opinion although never a final decision. My clients always seemed to me to be relieved that at least some measure of the responsibility for decision had been shifted from them. I often pointed out that the expectation of life for a canine or feline friend was only perhaps one seventh part of that of their owners. A parting, and often as not more than one, was inevitable.

Vivisection is a subject charged with much emotion by people, and suffering by animals. Certain advances in the study of medicine, surgery and pharmacology need to be monitored and assessed by the examination of their impact on live tissues. Remember though, that animals sometimes also benefit from such research. Procedures and drugs often extend their healing hand to animals as well as man. Vivisection should only be used only as a last resort. These animals are no mere chattels, but living things who like some soldier on the field of battle, unwillingly serve and often die. In many cases the attitude of people towards their fellow creatures appears of double standard, unbalanced, driven by emotion rather than compassion.

We hunt the fox to death but revere his close relative, the dog. We pursue the marlin and shark with ferocity and guile, but shed tears over a stranded whale or a netted dolphin. I watched a lady on television not long ago exhibiting a duck from whose feathers she had laboriously removed a clogging oil. She hoped the subject of her compassionate attention would be fit and well for the shooting season.

Animals suffer the unconscious cruelty of man, who sometimes perceive the animals they own as chattels satisfying some human need. But the animals are without a voice, unless perhaps in noisy or aggressive protest, and unable to state their case. The ravages of disease, flood and drought contribute enough to animal suffering without a man-made quota being added.

Animal welfare has made much progress in New Zealand but, as elsewhere, there is still some distance to travel. There is no more satisfactory affinity than that between man and mammals, but human appreciation, understanding, and perhaps education, is needed for this affinity to flourish. After all, man who has the casting vote.

Epilogue

After 40 years I wonder if I am better able to answer the query of my taxi driver in my first hour in the country when he asked, 'What do you think of New Zealand?'

Of course the question is hardly relevant, for the New Zealand of today is a place far different from the one I travelled to in the *Waiwera* in 1947. It is, I think, more sophisticated but less friendly. There are more rich and more poor. It is more materialistic, but not by much, and more emulative. It is more healthy but more stressed.

But I digress. Let me return to the question posed by my taxi driver. At the risk of being deemed repetitive and boring, I have to say that New Zealand is most likely the most beautiful country on earth. Mountain and river, meadow and coastline, combine in continuous panorama elsewhere unequalled. However these are fragile features which need a continuing vigilance for their protection. Luckily a relatively small population has had only comparatively few years to damage a sensitive environment, but within that time it has mounted a significant assault.

I recall a pleasant river near where I lived. It received the effluent from a large piggery, then the unwanted waste from a dairy factory. The freezing works made its obnoxious contribution before the now oily stream wound its way through a nearby township whose septic tanks had nowhere else for their overflow to go. This is still a major problem in large cities in which the sewage effluent from a large population is augmented by that from injudiciously sited freezing works. To this unsavoury bilogical emission is added an increasing volume of chemical waste, discharging eventually into water courses which find their way to the sea.

Many of New Zealand's unique plants, animals and birds have survived because no predators were present to interfere. But man, the greatest predator of all, soon put an end to this desirable co-existence. Rabbits, grazing even more closely than sheep, denuded steep slopes and so allowed topsoil to be washed into the valleys. Opossums, introduced to establish a fur industry, also acted as a reservoir host for bovine tuberculosis, an affliction not long ago near eradication. Rats threaten the survival of a number of native birds for they like to eat their eggs. Fast-flying aircraft offer possible haven to a large number of pests from other lands, mostly insects. Industrious officials, wielding their aerosol cans of insecticide when a plane from overseas arrives, may not prevent some of these from gaining a foothold.

As people and countries grow older and sometimes wiser, efforts to preserve what is important become more manifest. In places such as the high country, restoration may be difficult or even impossible. There is evident a stirring of conscience at most levels, and even if this is sometimes more emotional than practical we can indeed be thankful that it is there at all.

I have a pen pal in London — a lady with a skin of amber and a heart of gold. She writes, 'Why is it when your rugby teams — which usually win — are over here, before they play they sing a Maori song and do a Maori dance when most of them do not look like Maoris?'

It's not an easy question to answer and one which puzzled me when I first came to northern New Zealand. I discovered that some of the locals bore the same name as myself. They certainly did not look as if their ancestors had climbed the hills to the north of Loch Lomond as might have been expected of members of a sect of the clan MacGregor. It seemed as if some of my predecessors of earlier times had found romance and perhaps reward in the South Pacific to where they had sailed long ago. This racial confusion leaves me wondering if the word 'Maori' is now valid and is perhaps more a historical artefact to be preserved in that light. If, as many claim, we in this land are one, perhaps it is time to find a name applicable to all its inhabitants.

The name, of course, is already in place, so what of New Zealanders or Kiwis as they are sometimes called?

In sport they are certainly a remarkable lot, considering that the population is only a bit over three million. The Snells and the Walkers have run faster than the world's best. In rugby the feared All Blacks reign supreme. New Zealand yachts and horses traverse their respective elements faster than most, and when stumps are drawn an eleven from New Zealand has often proved itself at least equal to those from far more populous places.

I think that Kiwis are mostly achievers but the ones who lead have to be selected from the limited band of power seekers and are thus not those of the highest ability or intellect. This is a phenomenon by no means confined to New Zealand, but it perhaps explains why a country having unusually high natural resources in relation to the number of people who live in it does not always perform as well as it might.

I have noticed that Kiwis do not always have great respect for their bosses and this sometimes makes them poor employees. I think the instincts of the pioneer still shine through. I recall the fencers on my farm, the intrepid bulldozer driver carving a track on a precipitous hillside, the pilots with heavy load and little margin for error, giving life to flagging pastures. The Kiwi does best working for himself although sometimes betrayed by an ambition greater than judgement and energy greater than available capital input.

I think New Zealanders are a people of great tolerance and compassion; some would say to an extent which allows their leaders and, more especially sectarian groups, more latitude and privilege than they merit. The welfare state, at one time justifiably hailed as a prototype for all the world to follow, has become increasingly difficult to sustain. A population which had come to accept sustenance by the state as an unequivocal right now finds it increasingly difficult to adjust to the world of reality. I believe people are more appreciative by far if they have to work for their money and make provision for themselves but the transition for some may well be hard to bear. A few will always fall by the wayside and need aid from a compassionate state, but the need and the circumstances of origin should first be demonstrated.

I may well by now have answered at least in part the question my taxi driver back in 1947. If he is still around he may be disposed to add another, 'And how did you make out, mate?'

A good question, for achievement is more important than acquisition and contribution even more important than either.

I have, of course, established a new branch of the clan in a place far from Scotland's shores, and as the branch apparently continues to flourish I guess that that must be my highest accomplishment in a personal sense.

Nothing unusual in that I suppose, or in the daily efforts of a vet doing what he had been trained to do. There was a difference though, for I was a vet who trod where no vet had trodden before and a pioneer is always a bit unique.

I have been pleased to be associated with the control, if not the complete eradication of some of the great plagues of the animal kingdom. I believe that in the 1950's and 1960's more progress was made in this field than at any time before or since. This was especially so with hydatid disease. It can be clearly demonstrated that the benefit here positively flowed on to human health. Many people who are alive today would not be so blessed if the steps outlined had not been taken. With brucellosis vaccination through the years, followed eventually by blood testing, the incidence of abortion has been reduced to an insignificant proportion. Leptospirosis, if not completely controlled, has at least been identified and effective measures instituted and available to limit its spread. Bovine tuberculosis was all but eradicated when I hung up my boots and I hope that those in control today will not allow a resurgence and so negate the tiring and sometimes dangerous hours spent by many of my colleagues, operating in more ways than one in the testing times of the sixties.

In a personal sense, my thoughts often stray back to that land overlooked by the hills of Taiamai. I found it rewarding attending the sick and suffering, and for the most part earning the gratitude of patient and client alike. It was those same hills that overlooked the stony acres of our farm. I think we left those acres greener and more orderly than when we came, while their black and white inhabitants on two legs and four, went on to climb further mountains and find further rivers to cross.

> *If a guiding star you seek for life,*
> *Land or gold; husband, wife.*
> *Changing channels you may explore,*
> *But leave things better than before.*